An Orgasm (or More) A Day

AN ORGASM (or More) A DAY

365 WAYS to a *mind-blowing, deliciously satisfying, full-body orgasm*

REBECCA SWANNER
Former editor at *Penthouse*

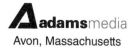

Avon, Massachusetts

Published by
Adams Media, a division of F+W Media, Inc.
57 Littlefield Street, Avon, MA 02322. U.S.A.
www.adamsmedia.com

ISBN 10: 1-4405-5094-8
ISBN 13: 978-1-4405-5094-2
eISBN 10: 1-4405-5095-6
eISBN 13: 978-1-4405-5095-9

Printed in the United States of America.

10   9   8   7   6   5   4   3   2   1

Contains material adapted and abridged from:
Oh My God! 365 Ways to Get Off by Rebecca Swanner, copyright © 2010 by F+W
Media, Inc., ISBN 10: 1-4405-0346-X, ISBN 13: 978-1-4405-0346-7; *The Everything*®
Orgasm Book by Amy Cooper, PhD, copyright © 2010 by F+W Media, Inc., ISBN 10:
1-60550-992-2, ISBN 13: 978-1-60550-992-1; and *The Everything*® *Great Sex Book,
2nd Edition* by Bobbi Dempsey, copyright © 2010 by F+W Media, Inc., ISBN 10:
1-4405-0148-3, ISBN 13: 978-1-4405-0148-7.

Interior illustration © istockphoto.com/Rapideye

*This book is available at quantity discounts for bulk purchases.
For information, please call 1-800-289-0963.*

Contents

Introduction

"An orgasm a day keeps the doctor away."

We can thank the seductive film actress Mae West for that great quote and she's right—orgasms are great for the mind, the spirit, and the body. They flood your brain with chemicals that make you happy, they help you connect with your lovers, and they may even help boost your immune system.

And, of course, they feel really, really, *really* good.

Many people view the orgasm as the ultimate goal of sexual activity, and that makes sense, right? You go through all the effort to get the pleasurable jolt at the end, but it's the journey to orgasm that makes it so good, not the orgasm itself. When you pay attention to your partner's (or your own!) deepest, darkest lusts, desires, and fantasies to take things deeper, harder, wetter, or faster, the erupting orgasm that follows is all the sweeter because of it. And that's what you are working toward here: finding new and interesting ways to *get* to orgasm.

In this book, whether you're a first-timer virgin or a seasoned expert who thinks you've tried it all in the bedroom, you'll find 365 tips that will help you experience orgasm (whether it's your first or thousandth), and then you'll learn how to take your orgasms from "meh" to *amazing*. And no matter how experienced you are, there are at least a few tips in here that will be new to you. So, what are you waiting for? It's time to get busy!

Ready to go? Grip your pillow tight, turn up the music, and get ready to orgasm like you never have before! Yes, yes, yes!

A Quick Note Before We Hit the Sheets

A note to those ladies who love women (or women and men): Throughout this book, for the purpose of clarity only, we refer to "your partner" as male and use a heterosexual relationship as the basis for the tips. In fact, there are even devoted sections called out as "For Him" so he can get in on the fun, too! However, this does not mean, in any way, that you shouldn't use the relevant tips to enjoy lovemaking with your female partner! In fact, please do! The more orgasms in the world, the better!

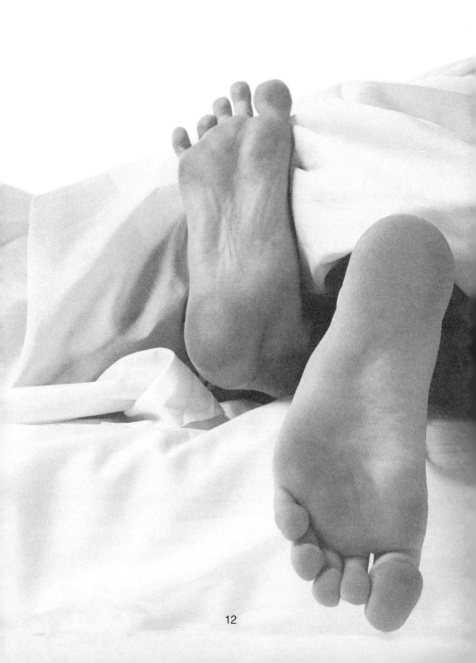

CHAPTER ONE

Orgasm by Knowing Yourself Intimately

1. Know Your Body—and His, Too!

When it comes to experiencing a powerful, memorable—and most important of all, repeatable—orgasm, the most important thing you can do is to get to know your body and become comfortable with it. No matter how intimate you become with your partner's— or partners'—body, you'll never be able to fully experience the wonder of an incredible orgasm without also becoming even more intimate with your own. After all, you're stuck with it your whole life—might as well love and enjoy it, right? In the chapter that follows, I'm going to take you on a tour of the female anatomy so that you have a solid foundation of your girlie parts before we move on to the really fun stuff. They say knowledge is power, and where better to have a little bit of power, if not in the bedroom?

So, you want to orgasm, huh? Like, *really* orgasm? Great! Before you get to the really fun stuff, it's important to review some basic anatomy. This way, when I suggest different parts of your partner's body—or your own—to stimulate in later chapters, you'll know just where to go. Plus, this brief review will help you become further acquainted, and more at ease, with the naughty bits, which will take some of the stress out of lovemaking and make it that much easier for you to have a mind-blowing orgasm. So bear with me for a moment and pretend you're in the best health class you never took. You'll thank me later.

2. Feel Good about Your Body

Before we delve into a deeper look at what's going on down below, let's take a more holistic look first. How do you feel about your body? Do you feel comfortable in your skin? Do you feel confident about certain parts but not others? Do you feel shy and uncomfortable or ashamed about your body in general? Notice your posture when you stand. Do you stand straight and tall with your chest up, or do you slouch with your shoulders drooping inward and your head down? Most likely you fall somewhere between those extremes, but it's important to realize that if you're closer to the latter than the former, you need to make some changes to become a more confident person.

When it comes to having a great orgasm, it's very hard to allow yourself to fully embrace the pleasure of the sensation if you don't feel confident about your body. As a woman in modern society, feeling totally confident about your body all of the time is unrealistic. Whether your source of discontentment comes from you holding yourself to the unrealistic standards portrayed in mass media (hello, Photoshop!), a not-so-nice partner (time to say bye-bye to that one about now), or something else that's rooted deeper, it's important for you to embrace the amazing goddess that you are. Own it, girlfriend. Seriously.

EXERCISE

I want you to do something for me. Go find a full-length mirror and stand in front of it naked. Yup, naked. Now, instead of focusing on what you've determined are "trouble spots," find at least three things you adore about your body. Anything goes, from your eyes to your hands to your stretch marks. Do this every morning until you start to think of yourself differently and focus on the positive aspects of yourself. Not only will this help make those "trouble spots" vanish from your vision, but you'll gain a lot more confidence in yourself both in and out of the bedroom. And how awesome is that?

3. Explore the Female Anatomy

While we're talking about mirrors, let's move on to discussing your anatomy down under. There's a lot going on under the surface of a woman, and I'm not just talking about your inner monologue. As you probably already know, unlike men, whose sex organs are external, your sex organs are located both on the surface of your body and inside of it. We're complicated like that. But it doesn't take a genius to learn how our different parts work, even if they're not as obvious as the male genitals. It just requires a little investigating. But it's fun investigating that can help lead to orgasm! So, go find a handheld mirror so we can begin exploring and learning about your amazing female anatomy. You'll be glad you did.

4. Press on the Pubic Mound

The pubic mound doesn't *sound* sexy, but it is. To get you oriented from an anatomical perspective, the pelvis bone wraps around your genitals and attaches your hips to your spine and to your legs. Atop of it is a mound of soft, fatty tissue known as the pubic mound, or *mons pubis*. It's located just above the Cleft of Venus, or Pudendal Cleft—known colloquially as the cameltoe. Men don't have this fatty mound, but during sex, yours is important to achieving a great orgasm because it protects you from bruising your pelvis, no matter how vigorously you're getting it on. In addition, some women can derive pleasure from their partner putting a significant amount of pressure on the pubic mound just before or during orgasm to heighten the sensation.

5. Get a Grip on the Lips

Below the pubic mound are the two softer vulva tissues known as the *labia majora* and *labia minora*, or "big lips" and "small lips." They begin at the Cleft of Venus and run parallel to the vaginal opening to the perineum, located just behind the vagina. The labia are similar in structure to the male scrotum, though they serve a different function. Whereas the scrotum helps to keep sperm at the optimal temperature, the labia protect the vaginal opening from bacteria. If you look, you'll easily be able to see the labia majora, as they are the larger structures. When pushed apart, you may be able to see the soft, delicate inner lips known as the labia minora, but sometimes these can be quite small. However, when you're aroused, these—like the clitoris—become engorged and are easy to find. Some women find that having these lips gently stroked during foreplay can be incredibly arousing and can help bring them to orgasm.

6. Awaken the Clitoris

Sometimes known as "the little man in a boat" or "the shining pearl," this tiny, roundish knob located at the top of the vulva, just above the urethra opening, is more than likely what holds the key to having an amazing orgasm. As far as scientists and anthropologists have discovered, the clitoris exists solely for sexual pleasure. Wahoo! And, though the entire clitoris is sensitive, the part of the clitoris with the most nerve endings per square inch is the glans. This is what you see when you pull back the clitoral hood that protects it from being touched directly. If this sounds at all familiar, that's because the clitoris is almost structurally identical to the penis. The glans of the clitoris corresponds to the glans of the penis, and the clitoral hood to the foreskin. However, whereas much attention is lavished on the shaft of the penis—or rather, how much shaft there is—this part of the clitoris is buried underneath the surface of the vulva (the collective name for all the external female sex organs in this area of your body). The clitoral shaft is attached to the pubic mound, is approximately one to two inches long and just over half an inch wide, and extends in two branches—called the *crura*—around the vaginal opening.

When you get turned on, the shaft becomes engorged with blood, and if you've ever felt a pleasurable throbbing around your vagina, this is the cause of it. Though as women we'll never understand just what a male erection feels like, I can imagine it's a similar sensation.

7. Delve Into the Vaginal Opening

I'm pretty sure you're familiar with the vaginal opening, but just in case, right below the urethral opening, you'll see the opening to the vagina—known in Latin as the *introitus* (feel free to drop that knowledge at your next cocktail party . . . or not).

When you're born, the vaginal opening is often at least partially covered with the hymen, a thin membrane that provides a barrier to protect the vagina from infection. And while the phrase "popping the cherry" still exists as a way to refer to losing one's virginity, a hymen can tear long before you ever have sex. It can be broken by the insertion of a tampon, finger, or sex toy, or even if you engage in activities like horseback riding. More than likely, the breaking of your hymen went unnoticed.

The vaginal opening is the narrowest part of the vagina, but this and the first internal third of the vagina itself together make up nearly 90 percent of the vagina's nerve endings! This is the primary reason why penis length, for the most part, doesn't matter. At the end of the day, it's more the girth—or circumference of the penis—that can make a difference in the intensity of orgasm. That said, you don't have to make love to a man who's particularly wide to enjoy a great orgasm. That's because during sexual activity, the vaginal opening will tighten as the nearby vestibular bulbs swell, and you'll feel the object inside of you that much more strongly. On the receiving end, your partner will feel a pleasurable gripping sensation. This gripping sensation can be further exaggerated for an even more profound orgasm, but I'll discuss that more a bit later.

8. Explore the First Part of the Vagina

For some women, this is where the magic happens. For others, the sweet spot is tied most directly to the clitoris or the vaginal opening. Sex—and orgasm—is all about personal preference, so it shouldn't be a surprise to find out that penetration is what works for some women but not for others.

Either way, the vagina is an integral part of your female anatomy, so let's take a moment to understand how it's designed. The vagina is a cylindrical, muscular structure that expands to its full potential when one is aroused. It's also able to stretch to accommodate large male members as needed. And, though it is just one structure, it has different textures. The outer third is composed of numerous ridges and folds and has more nerve endings than the rest of the vagina. And when you're aroused, the Bartholin's glands located near the opening of the vagina release a slippery fluid that lubricates the area and makes penetration easier.

9. Explore the Depth of the Vagina

As you go deeper into the vagina, you'll discover that the inner two-thirds are much smoother and less sensitive than the outer third. However, they do respond pleasurably to pressure. Finally, at the very end of the vagina is the cervix. This is the small tube through which sperm passes on its way into the uterus. Some women find it pleasurable when their cervix is bumped during sex, while others find that sensation wholly uncomfortable. You'll have to try a position that allows your partner to penetrate you deeply to find out which you prefer.

10. Discover the G-Spot and the A-Spot Pleasure Zones

I'm going to explore the G-spot, or Gräfenberg spot, and the A-spot in more depth later in the book, so for now, here are the basics. The G-spot is a mound of erectile tissue located two to three inches inside the vagina on the side facing the navel. When you're turned on, this area becomes engorged with blood and enlarges. If stimulated in a certain way, the Skene's glands located within it will ejaculate a clear or milky fluid. Yes, this is what has been nicknamed squirting.

Another sensitive location within the vagina is known as the anterior fornix erogenous zone, or the A-spot. This spot is located beyond the cervix where the vagina curves upward. The gland lubricates the vagina and, when stimulated, can deliver an intense orgasm.

11. Get Down with the Male Anatomy

Now that we've explored your anatomy, let's take a look at what the guys have going on. Unlike the female anatomy, the male sex organs—with the exception of the prostate—are all located on the outside of their body. And while each man has his own way he enjoys being pleasured, the easy access makes their anatomy a bit easier to find and stimulate.

Take a look at your partner while he is naked. Just like you, your partner should love his own body unconditionally—and you should love it, too. You will be in a much better place to give and receive orgasms from him if you do. Much like the earlier activity you did with your own body, look at your partner and make a verbal list of all the things you love about his body, whether it be the curves of his thighs, the smoothness of his hands, the length of his fingers, etc.—you may just orgasm right there, hearing all of his sexy attributes out loud!

12. Penis Play

Whereas women derive pleasure from stimulation of the labia, vaginal opening, vagina, and clitoris, men primarily derive pleasure from the stimulation of the penis. The penis is composed of three main sections: the shaft, the glans, and the corona glandis. On average, the erect penis is six inches in length and approximately five inches in circumference at its widest point. Interestingly, some men grow a lot in size from flaccid (or limp) to when they're fully erect, while others grow very little. Additionally, despite the claims of countless spam e-mails and Internet advertisements, it is not possible to enlarge the penis without undergoing cosmetic surgery. But you know the saying: It's not the size of the wave, but the motion of the ocean that matters when it comes to reaching orgasm.

13. Grip the Shaft

The shaft is made of three columns of spongy tissue—comparable to the tissue found in the clitoral shaft—that become engorged when a man is turned on and cause the penis to become erect and stand away from the body. When the penis is relaxed, or flaccid, the skin is loose and stretchy, which helps prevent it from becoming chafed during regular daily activities. But when it becomes erect, the skin becomes more taut and the shaft's sensitivity heightens greatly. One of the most sensitive areas on the shaft is known as the raphe. The raphe is a long line that runs up the shaft lengthwise and is filled with nerve endings. But, like with women and their sex organs, that may or may not work in turning on your partner, so make sure to play around and try all sorts of different touches and techniques to bring him to orgasm.

14. Tease the Glans

Sometimes referred to as the mushroom tip, this is the rounded part of the penis that is at the end of the shaft. It is developed out of the same tissue as the head of the clitoris, and as a result, for most men, this is an extremely sensitive area filled with many nerve endings. At the top of the glans lies the urethral opening through which both urine and semen are expelled, and just under the head of the glans is the frenulum. This frenulum is an area that is highly sensitive to touch. In uncircumcised males, this part of the penis connects to the foreskin and helps pull the protective hood over the glans.

But, you may still be wondering, why does it have that distinctive, mushroom-like shape? One theory is that the rounded head developed during human evolution so it was capable of pulling out any remaining semen from other males that had mated with the female so that their own sperm could impregnate her. In fact, across the animal kingdom, penises come in all shapes and sizes. But humans are the only species that have this mushroom cap. Another theory—which is not mutually exclusive—is that the mushroom shape increases friction and tension by stretching the vaginal opening, thus heightening female pleasure and the potential for orgasm.

15. Cue In on the Corona Glandis

This ridged "crown" of muscle—also sometimes referred to as the coronal ridge—is the part of the penis at the bottom of the glans. It is wider than the glans and any part of the shaft, and from an evolutionary perspective, it is the part of the penis responsible for collecting and removing the sperm of any competing male. But it is also extremely sensitive to the touch, as it is composed of thousands of nerve endings, and extremely sensitive to light touches, as well as pressure and temperature changes. To get your man hot and bothered, try stroking it lightly or exhaling, using your hot or cool breath to work him into a frenzy.

FUN FACT

Okay, size does matter a little bit. Men with longer penises are able to deposit their sperm further into the vagina (and closer to the cervix through which sperm can make their way to fertilize the egg) in a place where less well-endowed men would have a harder time scooping out their seed.

16. Feel the Foreskin

This small bit of skin—also known as the *prepuce*—is what covers the head of the penis and protects the urethra from bacterial infection when the penis is not erect. If you've lived in the United States your whole life, you might be surprised to discover that it is estimated that only one-sixth to one-third of the world's male population have had their foreskins removed in a surgery known as circumcision. Though in the United States it seems that circumcision is a customary procedure, despite its long-standing history (it dates back to at least the time of the Egyptians and is a commandment from God to those who practice the Jewish faith), it is not as popular around the world as you might believe. In fact, the act of circumcision has recently become a subject of debate in the United States as to what impact the practice has upon a child's emotional and psychological development, as well as the potential dulling of the glans.

Despite those concerns, if your partner is uncircumcised, you can help him to reach orgasm by running the foreskin back and forth over the glans of his penis, teasing him with that sensation.

17. Fondle the Scrotum and Testes

Below the penis lies the scrotum, the muscular pouch containing two sperm-producing, testosterone-making factories known as the testicles. Because the testes are very sensitive to touch and their ability to make healthy sperm is dependent on remaining at a temperature just lower than the male's internal body temperature, the scrotum raises and lowers the testes with the help of the cremasteric muscle. When it is too cold outside for the testes, the cremasteric reflex kicks in and the scrotal sac pulls the testes in toward the body; and when the body is very warm, it distends to let them cool off.

During oral or manual stimulation, run your hands gently over the scrotum and pull lightly on it to give your partner pleasure. You can also bite the skin gently, but be careful not to bite the testes themselves, as this could have quite the opposite effect that you were hoping for.

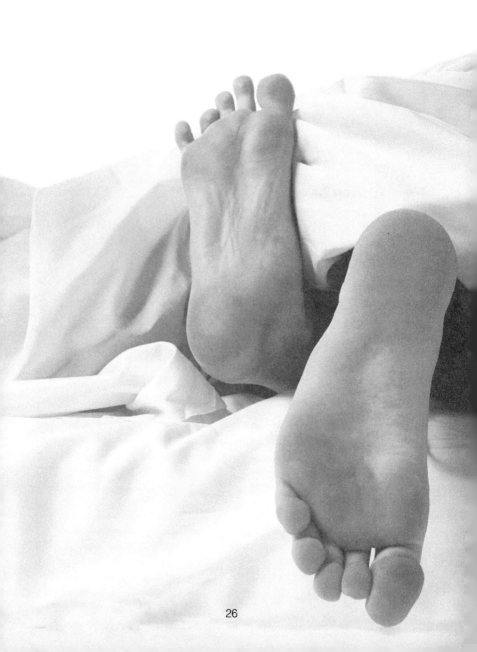

CHAPTER TWO

Get in the Erogenous Zone

18. Learn the Erogenous Zones

Now that you have a solid grip (ha ha ha!) on the male and female anatomy, it's time to move on to actually stimulating it so you—and your partner—can experience mind-blowing orgasms. One great way to begin to arouse each other is by stimulating each other's erogenous zones.

Have you ever felt the little hairs on your arms or on the back of your neck stand up when you're touched in certain places? That's probably because someone knowingly (or inadvertently) stimulated one of your erogenous zones. Named for Eros, the Greek god of love, these locations on the human body can trigger arousal when touched, kissed, licked, or stimulated in another way. There are two types of erogenous zones: specific and nonspecific. The specific ones include those that have mucous membranes. These include the lips, vagina, and penis. The nonspecific ones are those that are sensitive to touch but don't have mucous membranes, such as the scalp, underarms, and stomach. Because each person has his or her own favorite erogenous zones (as well as zones that may turn them off entirely), it's important to take the time to discover your and your partner's pleasure places. To get you started, here's how to stimulate those that are the most common.

19. Run Your Fingers Through His Hair

Ah, the scalp. The place from which all of your luxurious hair sprouts. Ever notice how relaxing it is after a long day to have someone play with your hair or massage your head? To take things to the next level and activate this secondary erogenous zone, gently massage the scalp with your fingers for a few minutes, making sure to cover the whole head—especially the extra-sensitive areas near the temples and behind the ears—and run your fingers through the hair. Pulling gently on a fistful of hair may also turn on those nerves and him with it. Then, have him do the same to you in return.

20. Nibble on the Ears

When done properly, ear play can arouse your partner to the point where they can't help but jump your bones. To get their fire started, place your index finger and thumb on opposite sides of their outer ear and slowly trace the edge of their ear from the top all the way down to the earlobe. Then, take the teasing play a step further by gently nibbling on and licking their earlobe. Try breathing softly around or into their ear or whisper some sweet nothings that only they can hear. If you're feeling particularly brave, you could use your tongue to circle their ear canal. For some, this is a serious turn-on, but for others, it can be a real turn-off . . . but hey, you never know until you try, right?

21. Activate Your Oral Stimulation

One of the greatest parts about kissing is that it stimulates the lips (and often tongues) of both partners! As you probably know, even kisses that involve just the lips can be a turn-on and can leave you wanting more. But kissing isn't the only way to activate his erogenous zone. Tease him by leaning over and slowly using your tongue to circle his lips, and forbid him to kiss you back if he tries to do so. Bite his lips gently and see how he reacts. As you slowly build up the tension, he'll be even more turned on when you finally lay a passionate one on him.

Another technique you might want to try when you're kissing him is running your tongue between the inside of your partner's lip and his bottom teeth. Just do it in a way that doesn't make him think you're fishing for the remnants of what he last ate.

22. Brush Against the Neck

Even if the recurrent vampire trends of the past decade haven't enticed you to want to start biting and sucking on necks, maybe the bloodsuckers of the night have the right idea. The neck has many areas that, when stimulated, can easily drive your partner wild. For one, start at the nape of your partner's neck and kiss them all the way down to their collarbone. Or, if your partner is more of the sensual variety, lick up one side of their windpipe and then the other with just the tip of your tongue and follow it by breathing over these same areas with your cold breath to ignite their senses. If he's more into the feel of your fingers, you can run your hands along his jawline, possibly even caressing his cheeks, and pull him in for a kiss.

Finally, if your partner is in fact into the sucking and biting-the-neck thing, do so, but begin gently. Most people don't have a high pain threshold; and while the vampires make chomping into someone's neck look sexy, your partner is more likely to respond with "Ow!" One trick to make biting the neck more likely to be pleasurable than painful is to not bite the neck itself. Instead, follow the curve of the side of the neck down to the fleshy part where the neck and shoulder meet. Grab onto a significant amount of this flesh with your teeth and bite here. By doing so, you'll be stimulating one of their pressure points and the feeling they get is likely to be one of dull, but somehow pleasure-inducing, pain. Just don't overdo it, as your lover might not appreciate going to work with a hickey.

23. Have Him Rub Your Shoulders

After a long day, almost nothing feels better than having your shoulders rubbed by your significant other while you sit and relax. Preferably it's by a roaring fire with a drink—hot cocoa, whisky, or wine—in hand. Relaxation is such an important step on the way to having an amazing orgasm. To help get you there, ask your partner to stimulate this erogenous zone by using his hands to gently caress your neck and shoulders in a circular motion. Or, if you prefer a more intense massage to get the day's kinks out, have him put a little extra pressure on your pressure points that are located on the back about two inches below where the side of your neck meets your shoulders. Perhaps these sensual activities will also encourage him to begin nuzzling your neck and kissing you all the way from your shoulders, across your collarbone, up your neck, and onto your lips. Still feeling stressed? I didn't think so.

24. Amp Up Arousal Through the Underarms

Though at first the underarms may seem like an odd erogenous zone, many women—and men—are turned on by having their underarms stimulated (note: I didn't say tickled). Not only do the armpits release powerful pheromones (these are the invisible chemicals that attract us to certain partners), but they are also filled with easily aroused nerve endings. When your partner is topless or wearing a sleeveless shirt (or if the whole sweat thing really bothers you, wait until they've just come out of the shower), lift up his arm and run the tips of your fingers down their underarm with just enough pressure so you don't tickle them. If your partner likes the sensation and you're feeling particularly adventurous, repeat the same motion, but with your tongue. You could even extend the movement from his wrist all the way down to his hips.

25. Use Your Breath to Electrify Your Lover

Partners who like their arms scratched, kissed, licked, or caressed will likely also enjoy having the inside of their elbows and wrists or the back of their knees stimulated. All of these areas are those where the skin is thin and it's easy to activate their nerve endings. That said, your partner might also be rather ticklish in these areas. To try and arouse without tickling, try licking then blowing your warm breath on them in a circular motion, before sealing the moment with a tender kiss. You can also try gently biting on these areas, but be careful—there might not be much to grab onto there!

26. Relax the Hands and Fingers

Hand massages are nice, particularly if you spend most of the day working with your hands. And considering that many of us have desk-type jobs, we do! Have your partner begin with the palm of your hand and gently massage your entire palm, as you navigate them with your oohs and ahhs. Then have them work their way up each of your fingers, relieving any tension you're holding in your digits. Return the favor for them, too. This may not be a direct gateway to having an incredible orgasm, but it is a way to help each other release the stress from the day and get on to the night's fun adventures.

27. Suck on the Fingers

A delicious, arousing technique is to suck on your partner's fingers or have him suck yours. One by one, take each of his fingers into your mouth and, holding the rest of the hand, slowly suck on them, stopping and flicking your tongue at the tip of the one you hold in your mouth. To him, if he submits to the pleasure, it might feel like you're going down on him . . . or it might lead things in that direction!

For an extra surprise, put a dollop of whipped cream or chocolate syrup on your finger to make your skin taste extra sweet. While he's working on your hand, feel free to take his other hand and put it to work on your favorite erogenous zone so you can get a doubly pleasurable experience. The wet sensation of his mouth on your finger coupled with the silky touch on your breasts, thighs, or clitoris can be just the ticket you need for a powerful, oh-so-yummy orgasm.

28. Love on the Breasts

Even if you're new to stimulating your or your partner's erogenous zones, I'll bet this is one you've already discovered. Most women love the feeling of their partner touching their breasts and nipples. As you may know, the sensitivity of your breasts may vary depending on where you are in your cycle and this can influence what sort of touch you find pleasurable. For instance, just before your period begins, they are likely to be super sensitive. During this time, you may find that you prefer your partner to be gentler with your nipples but a little more passionate with the larger part of your breasts. If your partner isn't sure where to begin, ask him to touch your breasts gently and start kissing and licking his way around them, starting from the outside of the breast and working his way to the center. Once there, ask him to slowly trace the outline of your areola and nipple with his tongue and lips, teasing you until you can't restrain yourself any longer.

Often, having your partner play with your breasts is a great lead-in to other forms of sexual play, but you might even discover that having your partner play with and suck on your breasts and nipples at certain times of your cycle is so stimulating that it could give you an orgasm on its own.

Though it might surprise you—and them—some men also have very sensitive breast tissue. While some men find having their nipples stimulated as exciting as hearing about the latest in celebrity gossip, flickering your tongue over the nipples and gently pulling on them with your teeth or fingers can drive others into a pleasurable frenzy. Try playing with his nipples and see what happens! You may awaken an erogenous zone your partner had not discovered!

29. Caress the Stomach

The way to the heart might be through the stomach, but it's also a pathway to orgasm. One of the reasons it's so important to become comfortable with your body—no matter what sort of shape you're in—is because the stomach is an erogenous zone that just begs to be stimulated. And if you're self-conscious about it, well, there goes a whole area that can help you reach orgasm. Don't worry about how you look—trust me, your partner thinks you look pretty damn sexy when you're standing there naked, ready to receive and give red-hot orgasms.

One great position to stimulate the stomach is from behind. Sit in front of him and gently lean back. This will not only give him access to your chest as well as your stomach (and other areas that you'll enjoy him fondling), the position will also create a sense of intimacy between you and help you to relax and let go of any feelings of self-consciousness. Have him trace his fingers from the top of your stomach to just above your pubic mound, over your hip bones, and back up to your chest again. It won't take too many of these teases before you're grabbing his hand and pulling it down just a little further . . . then further . . . then . . .

30. Run Your Tongue up the Spine

When it comes to appearance *and* the erogenous zones, it's easy to focus on the front of the body. It's what we're used to paying attention to, it's the side we usually engage in when we interact with someone, and it's the front of the body that provides us with the visual cues (via body language) about how someone feels about us. But let's take a walk around the other side of the body for a moment and pay attention to these often overlooked areas to help you and your partner achieve some amazing orgasms.

For starters, the back is full of nerves—after all, the interior of the spine is the location from where all nerves generate—so let's take advantage of this. Position yourself behind your partner and run your hands up their back, either in a massaging motion or in a more passionate, playful way. Don't be afraid to use your nails gently—or, depending on your partner's proclivities, not so gently. Then, start at your partner's sacrum (the small of the back) and use your fingers or tongue and hot breath to wind your way all the way up to the nape of his neck. You could also focus primarily on the sacrum by teasing it with your fingers and tongue in small circles. By the time you reach their hairline, they'll be tingling in a good way.

31. Make His Butt Tingle with Desire

Whether you have a round, juicy butt or one of the more slender varieties, it's undeniable that most men find a great-looking rear end a turn-on. And, as you may have surmised, it's also an erogenous zone. Later in the book, I'll detail spanking and other activities that feature the butt; but for now, here is one technique for you to try: When positioned behind your partner, run your hands from the bottom to the top of your partner's butt and follow this up with kisses. When you're done, playfully bite each cheek and work your way down to the backs of the knees or upward toward the neck. Your partner won't be able to stay still for long.

FUN FACT

Why are men attracted to the butt? One theory is that because estrogen causes women to store fat around their butt, hips, and thighs, curvy butts indicate a woman is fertile.

32. Scratch the Inner Thighs

If you began with the first erogenous zone I suggested at the top of your partner's body and are working your way down, by the time you make it to his inner thighs, he's likely to be very turned on and strongly wanting to move on from foreplay to more overtly sexual activities. If you're trying to go all the way—i.e., down to his feet— then just be ready for him to want to release his animal passion in the sack shortly thereafter. But for now, to set his inner thighs afire, begin by caressing his thighs with light, featherlike touches that come very near, but don't touch, his genitals. Slowly, get closer and closer to his penis and testicles and begin to incorporate kissing and added pressure to bring him to the breaking point.

33. Pay Attention to the Perineum

For those unfamiliar with this area, the perineum is the area between the vaginal opening and the anus on a woman, and between the testicles and anus on a man. While men often put some pressure on this spot during masturbation, it's an area that's often forgotten about when it comes to stimulating our partners. Ask him to gently massage this area either during foreplay or to turn you on even more when he's manually stimulating you to help you experience a more powerful orgasm. And when it comes to returning the favor, when he's near orgasm, push gently on this area to heighten the explosion.

34. Touch the Toes

There's a reason Samuel L. Jackson's character in *Pulp Fiction* believed that Marsellus Wallace had a guy knocked off a roof for massaging his wife's feet. Having your feet rubbed feels good. Really good. This is especially true if you're the type who loves to wear heels or your partner regularly wears dress shoes. Because whether or not you want to go a step further and experiment with putting your partner's toes in your mouth, which to some is a serious turn-on, a gentle foot massage is sure to make your partner feel completely relaxed—especially if you're kind enough to first soak the feet in a tub of warm water or the bath. And, as you've learned, relaxation is a crucial pathway to having a great orgasm.

But massaging the feet isn't just about relaxation. Reflexologists believe that by massaging different areas of the feet (or hands), you can help heal other ailments in the body, and supposedly, putting extra pressure on the bottom of the sole (near the heel) will arouse the sex organs. Just don't do this to someone else's husband (or wife) unless you're ready to pay the consequences.

35. Connect Your Erogenous Zones to Your Genitals

You and your partner will likely discover that touching the erogenous zones I've outlined within this chapter feels amazing. But to make them feel that much *better*, try—in your mind—to connect them to your genitals. This way, when these areas are stimulated, they have that much more power to turn you on and get you closer to orgasm. When you're on your own, pick one of your favorite erogenous zones to stimulate. As you touch this area and become more turned on, notice the throbbing in your genitals. Then, as you continue to touch this erogenous zone, shift your attention back to that area and imagine that, say, as you are stroking your stomach, you're actually running your fingers over your clitoris. By mentally connecting your erogenous zones with your genitals, you'll find it easier to become aroused and with enough practice, the simple touches your lover delivers will leave you eager for more.

> ### FUN FACT
> Your whole body is one big erogenous zone. Touch applied to your hair follicles and nerves on the skin travels to the brain and is translated to erotic, sensual feelings of pleasure. But some areas are more sensitive

than others, so your body's erogenous zones can generally be divided into three different types:

1. **Primary (first-degree) erogenous zone.** These include the mucous membrane tissues that comprise the lips, genitals, and nipples. These areas include the anus, penis, vaginal lips, and inside the outer third of the vagina. They are rich in nerves and the nerve endings are very close to the surface of the skin. These areas are very responsive to touch.

2. **Secondary (second-degree) erogenous zone.** Parts that have a sparse amount of hair and are often found in the regions next to the third-degree areas. These parts are not as sensitive as the primary erogenous zone, but are more sensitive than the areas covered by hair.

3. **Tertiary (third-degree) erogenous zone.** The areas of the skin that are covered with hair—your arms, legs, parts of the chest, and so forth. These areas have fewer and more dispersed nerve endings, so they are the least erogenous. Nevertheless, the hair follicles' ends, down under the skin, help stimulate the nerve endings that are buried near them.

Of course, it seems obvious to go right for the first tier of these zones; but rather than reaching for your partner's genitals straight off the bat, try something new. By working on your secondary and tertiary erogenous zones, you are training your body to feel much more. After some practice, it is even conceivable to reach orgasm just by having your nipples sucked. The possibilities are endless!

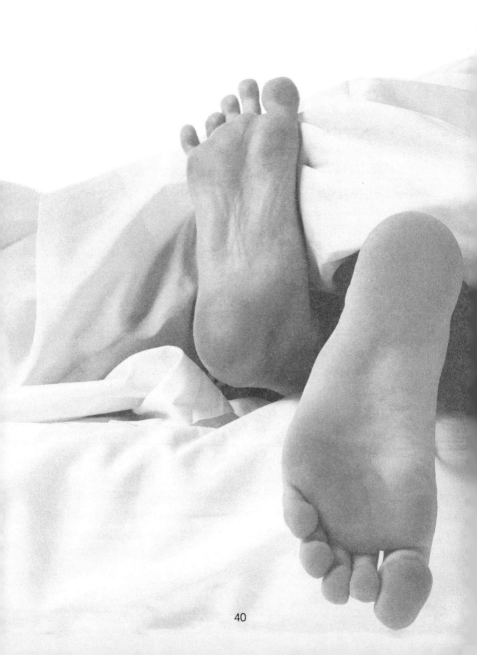

CHAPTER THREE

Get Your Body Ready

36. Understand What an Orgasm Is

Sometimes, understanding something can help us to experience it at a deeper level. So while all this talk about anatomy and your erogenous zones might have gotten your wheels spinning, you might still be wondering just exactly what is an orgasm? Even if you've had one—or many—you might not be able to explain that powerful, dramatic, explosive moment that's been dubbed the big O or, my personal favorite, *la petit mort*.

FUN FACT

The French phrase *la petit mort* translates literally to mean "the little death," but it's also an idiom for orgasm. But why? There are two schools of thought on this. One is that the phrase—which had its heyday in French literature during the late 1800s and early 1900s—refers to the blacking out/loss of consciousness feeling you experience during a powerful orgasm. During orgasm, the breath becomes more rapid and for some, this can cause hyperventilation and even fainting! Quick, fetch the smelling salts and loosen that corset!

Another possibility is that because cultures were once very concerned about the loss of any type of fluids from the body (and the body's balance of the fluids), every orgasm (and subsequent ejaculation) meant that you lost a bit of your life force. This idea dates at least as far back as the Bible, when God killed Onan for wasting his seed (sperm) on the ground.

An orgasm is, strictly speaking, the moment of sexual climax when certain muscle contractions occur and the heart rate, blood pressure, and respiration rate increase. There are all types of orgasms: ones in which men and women ejaculate and ones where they don't; ones that last a few seconds, ones that last much longer, and ones that happen over and over again; ones that result from clitoral stimulation; and ones that result from vaginal or anal stimulation, or even no stimulation at all!

Over the next few points, I'll explain how the human sexual response cycle works (or, in other words, how we get aroused). If you've been having difficulties reaching climax, this knowledge can help you understand where you're getting "stuck" and help you figure out how to reach the next step.

37. Orgasms Are Good for You

Several recent studies point to the slew of great health reasons to get busy—often! Aside from the cardiovascular benefits of sex, research shows regular sex and orgasms can provide migraine relief and stress relief, help you sleep deeply, boost immunity and self-esteem, alleviate pain associated with PMS, and protect against prostate and other cancers and heart disease. Not that I thought you really needed more reasons to have sex, but in case you did—just remember that regular sex does a body good!

38. Get a Grip on Your Cycle

Though not impossible, it is difficult for two adults to have sex with one another if neither is aroused. Should the man even be able to penetrate the woman, there would be so much friction within her vagina that the resulting sex would be terribly uncomfortable.

But as we become aroused, our bodies experience certain physiological changes and react in specific ways that make having sex easier (and much more pleasurable). After observing the changes in 382 women and 312 men during sexual activity, sexologists William H. Masters and Virginia E. Johnson divided the different physiological changes the body experiences into the excitement phase, plateau phase, orgasmic phase, and resolution phase. The results were published in their 1966 book *Human Sexual Response*. Since the publication of their research, a fifth stage, desire, has been added to the forefront of the cycle. Read on to learn what these stages are and how you can use them to double your pleasure.

39. Acknowledge Your Desire

Desire is the first step that kicks off the sexual response cycle. This urge for sexual intimacy or gratification mostly occurs in the mind. Before a penis begins to get erect or your vagina starts to become lubricated, an enticing thought or someone in your view must ignite your internal fire. It might be someone who has just come into view, your partner, an image on a screen, enticing words on a page, or even just a hot thought that passes through your mind. Especially because desire is entwined with memory, it can be ignited by any of the senses. For instance, if you catch a whiff of cologne in the air, it could spark your desire if someone you used to have a romantic interest in used to wear it. But desire can also be negatively affected by feelings of low self-esteem, intense stress, poor health, low energy, and—depending on what time of the month your menstrual cycle is in—hormonal levels. There's a reason why I've been reminding you again and again how important feeling confident in your skin and being relaxed in the bedroom are to achieving a powerful orgasm. When those two factors are out of balance, you erect a barrier to jump-starting your sexual response cycle.

40. Get Excited

The second step in your sexual response cycle is excitement. This occurs when you've begun to act on your initial impulse of desire and have started to physically sense arousal within your body.

It's at this time that heart rate speeds up, the breath quickens, and the muscles become tenser, especially around the genitals. There is also an increase in blood flow throughout the body, and this may result in the torso or face becoming flushed. Has there been a time when you and your partner were hooking up discreetly but were interrupted, and someone asked you why your face or chest was so red? Blame the "sex flush." When you're in this excitement phase, your nerves also operate slightly differently, as you are more sensitive to pleasure and less sensitive to pain.

You might notice your nipples becoming hard. But that's not all that's swelling. In men, the penis becomes erect, the scrotum thickens, and the testicles rise up closer to the body. In women, the clitoris, vagina, and vulva become engorged with blood, and the breasts might increase in size. It's also at this time that the vaginal walls become lubricated (also known as "getting wet"), the vagina lengthens, the upper portion of it expands, the uterus rises, and the labia swell and separate in expectation of penetration. As the desire phase prepares the mind for intercourse, the excitement phase prepares the body for sex.

41. Hit the Plateau

As with most things, you can't just continue along the same path forever. You can't just keep getting more and more excited. Eventually, you'll hit a plateau. This plateau marks the third step of your sexual response cycle and it is the step just before orgasm. It is often reached through continuous physical stimulation of erogenous zones or mental stimulation. It is also possible to slip from this stage back to the excitement phase (and return to the plateau stage again) multiple times up until the point of orgasm.

During this stage, many of the body's muscles have tensed, breathing rate and heart rate have quickened even more than in the excitement phase, and blood pressure levels have continued to rise. You may experience muscle spasms in your feet, hands, or face. Women experience the "orgasmic platform" during which the lower third of the vagina swells, tightens, and narrows, and the upper two-thirds expand further. Though this makes penetration slightly more difficult—but likely, more pleasant—the purpose of this orgasmic platform is so that the vagina can better catch any sperm that is released by the man during orgasm.

FUN FACT

Despite everything you've heard, it is not possible to get pregnant from pre-come. Recent scientific studies have revealed that most pre-ejaculate fluid (pre-come) does not contain sperm. If it does contain sperm, the sperm are immotile or dead. However, if your significant other does ejaculate a bit before pulling out, that can get you pregnant.

In addition, your vagina becomes even more lubricated, your nipples stand up, the areolae darken in color, and the clitoris becomes extremely sensitive to touch and hides for cover underneath its hood. In men, the penis becomes fully erect, and the glans swells to its largest size (in order to be most effective at pushing out any sperm it may encounter within the vagina). The testicles become fifty percent larger than they were prior to the initiation of the sexual response cycle, and the Cowper's glands will release viscous, pre-come fluid to clear the urethral tract of any residual urine that will kill sperm.

42. Hit Your Peak

This, step four of the sexual response cycle, is the moment you've been waiting for: the climax. It is during this phase that you experience the involuntary muscle contractions within your vaginal walls and men experience ejaculation. (It is, in fact, possible for you to ejaculate—or, to put it into the parlance of our times, to squirt—and I will cover how to do this later in the book). Immediately following this release, the brain instructs the body to flood the bloodstream with pleasure-causing chemicals known as endorphins, including but not limited to, oxytocin. The combination is what causes an orgasm to feel really, really good.

FUN FACT

As you probably know, some orgasms feel better than others. An orgasm's intensity is tied to the amount of oxytocin in the bloodstream. Oxytocin stimulates muscle contractions, so the greater the amount of oxytocin, the more powerful the release.

43. Take It Down a Notch

Following the fury of orgasm, resolution is the fifth and final step of the sexual response cycle. During this stage, the muscles that had been tensed relax, and breathing, blood pressure, and heart rate return to their original, nonaroused states.

For men, this stage also incorporates the refractory period, during which time it is very difficult, if not impossible, to experience a second orgasm and the penis might be extremely sensitive —possibly even painful—to touch. That is because the male body is processing the pleasure-inducing hormone oxytocin, but more importantly it is also processing the hormone prolactin, which depresses sexual arousal.

Some women also experience a refractory period, though others are able to have multiple orgasms before advancing to the resolution stage.

44. Create an Arousal Map

Now that you are familiar with the stages of the sexual response cycle, it is time to put your knowledge into action so you can determine what triggers your desire and sets the wheels of your cycle into motion. To do so, it can help to build an arousal map so you are more aware of your sexual triggers. Should you reach a time in your life when you're having a difficult time becoming aroused— whether this is due to boredom in a relationship, stress, or general lack of sexual desire—you can refer back to this collected list of ideas, thoughts, movements, smells, visual cues, etc., of what works for you to get out of your sexual rut. To begin, take out a piece of paper and ask yourself the following questions:

- When have you felt the most desire or pleasure?
- What places and times of day have turned you on the most?
- What partners have turned you on the most, or which ones did you feel the most sexually compatible with? Why?
- How is your sexual life similar or different now?
- What turns you on?

- What turns you off?
- How would you set up a sexual scene for yourself?

45. Create an Arousal Flow Chart

Now that you've created your arousal map, you should have a clearer idea of what turns you on and be aware of what challenges you need to overcome so that you can enjoy a fuller, freer orgasm.

Now you're going to build a chart of erotic stimulation that you or your partner can follow with the purpose of causing you to have an amazing, mind-blowing orgasm. Building this chart is going to be easy and fun.

Start by caressing different areas of your body to see which ones spark the most erotic sensations. It's not cheating if you start with your genitals, but try to think a *little* outside the box, hmm? If you're stuck, refer back to the erogenous zones you recently learned about, but also explore everywhere on your body you feel might turn you on. As you begin to turn yourself on, take mental notes of which areas spark the most desire and in which order. Should your partner play with your entire torso for a few minutes, then progress to caressing your neck before moving on to licking your inner thighs? If you're able to write all of this down while pleasuring yourself so you have these thoughts to refer back to later, even better.

Once you've experimented with different sequences (this will likely require more than one session), put this flow chart into play when you're masturbating or with your partner and see if it works. Make adjustments as you need to, as this is a great chart to return to when you're sexually unsatisfied.

By knowing what sort of attention your body requires to reach each stage of the sexual response cycle, you're putting the key to having a successful orgasm in your hands and you'll be that much more likely to experience a great one.

46. Relax

While an orgasm may release some of your stress, if you're tense prior to lovemaking, it's going to be much harder to "get there." Before you engage in sexual play, try to take your mind off of what is causing your stress or do something that will release your stress altogether. Exercise. Take a hot bath. Watch television. Play a video game. Knit. Meditate. Exercise (this is such a powerful tool for taking your mind off of what is bothering you that I'm including it twice). Entering into lovemaking relaxed will result in a more fun session and, likely, a more satisfying orgasm.

47. Breathe

When we are stressed or anxious, we often don't take full breaths—and this makes it harder to have a great orgasm. When you're feeling tense, your breaths are likely to be much shorter than they are when you're relaxed. One excellent way to start to relieve stress is with deep breathing. Those who do yoga on a regular basis are familiar with this style of breathing, but if it's been a while since you've done the downward dog, let me guide you. First, lie down and get comfortable. Then place one hand on your abdomen and practice filling this up with a breath. As you do, that area will expand. Slowly count to ten as you inhale, then hold for five counts, then exhale for ten counts. If that is too difficult, start with five or seven counts, but try to keep your mouth closed and breathe through your nose. Once again, if this is too difficult, start by breathing in through your nose and out through your mouth. But whatever you do, breathe slowly using your abdomen, not your chest. As you practice calm, mindful breathing, you will find yourself slipping into a calm, meditative state. This is great not only for helping you to achieve a better orgasm, but also to find calm in stressful situations (traffic, work meetings, etc.).

48. Meditate

Not only is meditation a great way to relax and center yourself, it is also a great way to focus your mind. When you're in the mood for sex or sexual activity but a million things are going through your mind—what to do for dinner, how to deal with your roommate, what to do with the kids, the latest drama at work—it helps to shut off all those thoughts, quiet your mind, and put your attention on the matter at hand, namely, the hot person you want to make love to who is sitting in front of you. There are many types of meditation, but here is a simple one to get you started. This one can be done at any time of the day and for any length of time. Begin by breathing deeply. Once you are in a calm state, begin to focus on your breath. As thoughts come up, do not follow them. Do not worry about not following them. Just continue to focus on your breath as you allow your mind to quiet. Try to remain in this meditation for at least five minutes.

49. Eat Right

Eating right is so important. Not only do light, healthy meals make you more in the mood for sex (honestly, all I want to do after inhaling a burger and fries is sleep), but also eating nutrient-dense food provides your body with more useful energy than junk food (i.e., sugar-laden products) does. If you sense that your eating habits are suspect, consider starting a food diary to keep track of what you're really ingesting throughout the day and replace as many of the unhealthy choices with healthy ones as you can. Though it may be difficult at first, you'll find that the more fruits, vegetables, lean proteins, and whole grains you eat and the less processed food and refined sugar you digest will result in a you that has more energy for physical activities, including sex.

50. Take a Mental Health or Personal Day from Work

If you're like most people, nothing causes you stress like your job. So if you're sick and tired of working—or thinking about work—when you could be climaxing, take a personal day or call in sick. Take the day off to do some nice things for yourself and whittle down that to-do list that has been hovering in the back of your mind even when you're in the throes of passion. If your partner is able to take a day off as well, take advantage of it. Have sex in every room: missionary in the master bedroom, woman-on-top in the kitchen, doggie style in the den. Be as loud and as uninhibited as you can. Start at the crack of dawn, and have sex throughout the day. Begin with a hot wake-up call (foreplay for breakfast). Break for lunch (chocolate sauce, whipped cream, and him). Indulge in a little love in the afternoon (a little tantric sex, perhaps). Finish off with an Orgasm Contest, in which you challenge each other to achieve your own respective personal best climax counts. If you're experiencing your day off solo, that's okay too! Just make sure to also enjoy the pleasure of your own company!

51. Exercise

Exercise is another way to boost your sex life and your orgasm potential. Exercise causes your body to release feel-good chemicals known as endorphins, and we all know we're more in the mood to hop into bed when we're feeling confident about our bodies. The American Council on Exercise recommends twenty to thirty minutes of moderate exertion a day and claims that being at least this physically active can have results similar to taking Viagra.

On top of that, exercise can help you become more limber and agile . . . and you can only imagine how this can help in the bedroom. After a few months, or even weeks, at the gym, you'll start to notice that you can do things you couldn't do before—lift more weight, run longer, touch your toes. In addition, you'll probably literally be breathing easier. Aerobic exercise will build up your endurance so you'll have more stamina in the bedroom. That's sure to put a smile on your face and your partner's.

52. Try Yoga

Over the last few decades, yoga has really taken a hold in the Western world, and now, even if there isn't a dedicated yoga studio near your home or office, most gyms offer yoga classes. Those who engage in the practice regularly swear it has stress-reducing, life-enhancing effects, including flexibility. If there's a sexual position you've seen in a book or magazine that you want to try but you just don't think you're quite flexible enough, try indulging in yoga once or twice a week for a few months. You just might be closer to making that position happen. And those of you who are single might end up meeting another flexible soul in the process.

In addition, some moves open up the hip flexors to make certain positions easier while others, like the cat stretch, help strengthen the Kegel muscles. These muscles in your vagina allow you to grip the penis more tightly during sex and they're also the same muscles that shudder during orgasm. By strengthening these, you can help yourself achieve a more powerful climax.

53. Don't Censor Yourself

Do not worry that your sexual thoughts might be "wrong" or "weird." Everyone has different sexual proclivities and what may seem "odd" to one may seem "normal" to another. As long as your sexual desires do not cause another harm, do your best not to judge your thoughts. And remember, everyone has their "thing." Your fantasy does not hurt or objectify others, so it's fine.

If you can't shake the feeling you're being judged or that your thoughts are improper, here's another perspective for you to consider: If you have a fantasy that you think might be looked down upon, isn't it better to act out this fantasy in the safety of your own home with an understanding, consenting adult than to chide yourself for merely thinking it?

54. Banish Shame

Shame and fear are major mood killers and they can make it very difficult for you to reach orgasm. They also present themselves in various forms. If you are having difficulty getting past sexual shame or fear of your fantasies, these mindsets can very well be preventing you from having an amazing orgasm. Try, perhaps with the help of an objective, unbiased professional, to address the root cause of these feelings. Did your family, religion, culture, or past sexual experiences leave you with a negative view of your sexuality? Did you receive too little or not the right kind of touch growing up? Do you have low self-esteem or just a generally bad impression of yourself? Once you've discovered the reasons that have caused your misperception of sexuality, begin to work through—and release— these negative, self-restricting thoughts and resulting behaviors so you can enjoy a rich sexual life. If you've held onto these beliefs for a long time, don't expect your attitudes to change overnight, but with patience they will.

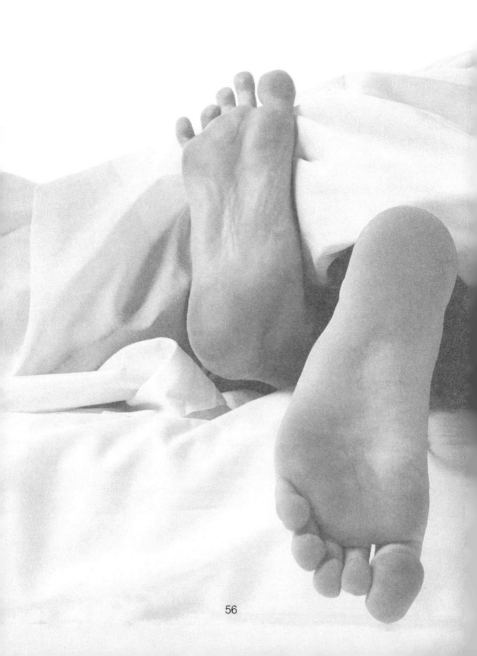

CHAPTER FOUR

Set the Scene

55. Set the Scene for Love

When it comes to having sex or making out, it's important to create a space that is welcoming to love. Small changes in your environment will heighten your mood, help you relax when you're in your home, and set the scene for the big O. To begin this process, work on reducing the amount of clutter in your home. Coming home to a stack of bills on the kitchen table and then tripping over dirty laundry and toys won't help you get in the mood. And, even if you *do* manage to get in the mood, you're likely to have trouble focusing on lovemaking when there's an insurmountable to-do list surrounding you.

So, if there's clutter peeking out from the cabinets and your surfaces are buried in papers and other items, it's time for a spring cleaning, even if it's the middle of November. If tidying your entire house feels too daunting, then just focus on the bedroom so you can have at least one sanctuary to retreat to. Remove misplaced items from surfaces, floor spaces, and closets and help them find a home. Put anything that is still usable but that you don't personally use or want into a box to donate, and remove excess furniture to make rooms feel more open. Then, clean. When you're done with this, your living space will feel fresh and inviting and help you to be more in the mood for something special to happen.

56. Transform Your Bedroom with Feng Shui

Even if you're doubtful about your interior decorating skills and are skeptical about Feng Shui, you can still utilize the traditional Chinese tool as a way to improve the flow of your home and the rooms within it. Feng Shui means "wind water" and is an ancient Chinese art and science that influences the direction of energy known as *qi* (pronounced "chee") within a space. The flow of the *qi* depends on the design of a building as well as the arrangement of objects within it. Whether or not you believe this is possible, some classic Feng Shui tips can help rooms—especially your bedroom—feel more inviting. Here are some easy and inexpensive ways to improve your bedroom that may help you to have a more powerful orgasm.

1. Remove plants, office equipment, exercise equipment, and the television from your bedroom.
2. Remove photos of friends and family as well as anything you're still holding onto that relates to former lovers from your bedroom. Do you really want your mother watching you make love? I'll let you answer that one.
3. As often as you can, keep your windows ajar to keep the air circulating.
4. Display only positive images and those that inspire love within your bedroom. Sorry, but that means your Slayer poster has to be moved to another room.
5. Position your bed so it is approachable from both sides and sits as far away from the door as possible. Avoid having the foot of it directly facing any door, including that of your closet.
6. Place nightstands on either side of the bed.
7. Remove objects from underneath the bed.
8. Give your bed a headboard. Even if it's one that's just painted onto the wall.
9. Place something that will make you smile directly in line with where you stand when you open the door so that every time you enter the bedroom, it will bring a smile to your face.

57. Make Your Bedroom a Sacred Space

Your bedroom is where two things should happen: sex and sleep. And, on occasion, breakfast in bed. It shouldn't be your second office, home gym, or where you watch television until you zonk out. Bringing those activities into the bedroom can make it harder for you to sleep peaceably and for lovemaking to happen. But by dedicating the space to these two activities and thus training your brain to associate only those activities with it, you'll know that whenever you're in the bedroom, it's to engage in one of two acts. To keep your bedroom a place where you go to get away from it all, do your best to not bring work into the bedroom or use the surfaces in the room to pile up things that have to be taken care of. If you have a walk-in closet, use that as your dressing area. Of course, depending on your living situation—for instance, if you live in a studio apartment or dorm—it may not be possible to devote your bedroom solely to these two activities. If that is the case, section off an area where you engage in other things with the help of a curtain, bookcase, or screen.

58. Make a Playlist

To set the mood, sometimes you need a little mood music. Go through your music library and pull together a playlist of songs that will enhance future lovemaking moments. If you're feeling stuck or aren't familiar with today's popular bands, sign up for Pandora or Spotify. Both services have a free option and can be used as tools to expand your musical knowledge. Just plug in the name of a band you do like and they will present you with a radio station based on that artist as well as a list of related artists.

I recommend that you put together a few playlists, as sometimes you'll probably want a slow, romantic night and sometimes you'll want to tear your lover's clothes off and drag him into the bedroom. If you prefer CDs or vinyl to the compressed sound of digital recordings, then burn a CD or put together a stack of LPs that would be perfect for each occasion and place them by the CD or record player so you don't have to fumble for them when you're on your way to a great orgasm.

59. Use Romantic Lighting

Mood music is important when it comes to setting the scene and pace for lovemaking, but mood lighting is critical to creating a sensual space. Unfortunately, we tend to think about lighting a room from a utilitarian perspective. We think about what light fixtures will create the *most* light in a room, not what *type* of light to create.

When trying to create a cozy, comfortable space, stay away from bright ceiling lights, as these can make whomever is on the bottom feel as if they are being interrogated mid-coitus. Instead, purchase lamps that create tantalizing shadows across your body. If you still need bright lamps to read or dress by, place these on the nightstands so you can turn them off without having to get out of bed in case the mood changes from relaxation to play. To help this to happen, I encourage you to keep at least one sexually stimulating book within reach of the bed. Even a discreet one—like the erotic tales by Anaïs Nin—will do the trick when you want to encourage yourself or your partner to get in the mood.

60. Live by Candlelight

Candles are one of the most sensual types of lighting you can employ. They come in all shapes and sizes, from small tea lights to enormous pillars, and are available in a variety of scents. If you are going to use scented candles, select ones that give just a hint of aroma to the room so you don't overpower the nose of you or your lover. Here are some scents that scientists have found to be effective at improving blood flow to the penis and causing arousal:

- Cinnamon
- Vanilla
- The combination of jasmine and rose
- Lavender
- Pumpkin pie

Of course, never leave an unattended candle burning. You want to light the flames of love, not burn the house down, so make sure to snuff out the flames before curling up into your lover's arms for some zzz's.

61. Get Great Sheets

Are you still using your old college sheets? If you're no longer in college and they're still in good condition, it's time to clean these with color-safe bleach and promptly donate them. The goal is to achieve amazing orgasm after orgasm, and as the primary space for this activity is your bed, it's important to outfit it properly with a quality mattress and luxurious sheets. Think about it: If you wanted to excel at running, you wouldn't train in your flip-flops, so stop having sex on uncomfortable sheets.

When replacing your old standbys, opt for something that feels sensual to the touch. Silk and satin are classic sexy options, but they're also not the most practical. They're difficult to keep clean and while they are easy to move around on top of, you might find they're a little *too* slippery. Instead, try Egyptian cotton sheets. Not only are they durable, they're also easy to wash and last longer.

Select colors that complement your skin tone or your eyes so you look even more ravishing when you're lying on them. Oh, and don't feel you need to throw umpteen pillows on the bed to make it look cozy. They'll just be more things to move out of the way when you want to start fooling around.

62. Get Off on Color

Color can have a profound impact on your mood, your ability to relax, your energy level, and your orgasm. Here's a brief rundown on what psychological effects different hues can have so you can select the one that is best for your bedroom needs.

1. Red—Shades of red stimulate the senses, but can heighten energy levels and make it difficult to fall asleep.
2. Blues and Greens—These colors cause us to feel calm and at peace. They're a great choice for the bedroom, though they may make some feel a little too relaxed.
3. Browns—This earth tone inspires coziness and connection with others.
4. Greys—As a psychologically neutral color, grey can inspire sensuality or it can dampen the mood.

If you're not up for repainting, you can also introduce splotches of color by reupholstering a chair, purchasing a rug, or replacing your old comforter cover with one in a new shade.

63. Create an Enticing Pathway to Love

If you're anticipating or planning a special night, take the time to not only transform your bedroom, but also to make the pathway leading to it a little more fun so your partner knows that something extra exciting is coming their way. Have that playlist you created a few tips ago playing softly when your partner arrives. Have a glass of wine or champagne waiting for each of you in the bedroom and leave a sex toy or two within view. (A tip for my male readers: Buy a small bouquet of roses and use it to sprinkle rose petals all the way down the hallway and onto the bed. It's an inexpensive touch that will absolutely be noticed.) If you tap into what your significant other finds romantic when you're picking out elements for the rendezvous ahead, you're sure to help each other down the path toward a great orgasm and a memorable night.

64. Be Aware of Your Surroundings

You've worked hard to transform your home and bedroom into an inviting, sensual sanctuary. Make sure to take the time to appreciate it. Use the tools I've taught you to really take it all in. Smell the scents. Fall in love with the color and the cozy, comforting aesthetic. Run your hands over the new sheets. Then make a date with your partner—or yourself!—to *really* enjoy your new surroundings.

65. Build Intimacy

Unless the type of sexual relationship you are currently looking for involves a one-night stand or a friend with benefits, it will absolutely help your sex life to work toward developing a deeper level of intimacy—or closeness—with your partner. Doing so will help you to feel much more at ease in the bedroom and more open to confessing your desires to your partner. It will also help you feel more comfortable leading them down the right path when they're not performing quite to your orgasmic satisfaction. Start by asking your partner what he considers intimacy to be—is it strictly a level of comfort, or something more? His answer could surprise you.

66. Be an Active Listener

One key aspect to feeling close with your partner—which can raise your oxytocin levels, and with them, the powerfulness of your orgasm—is to feel as if you two are communicating well. As you probably know, just because there are seemingly countless ways to communicate with your partner—to name just a few, there's texting, e-mail, online chat, Skype, Facebook, Twitter . . . and actually calling one another—that doesn't mean you're communicating well. If you find you have a habit of not actually listening to your partner but rather waiting to speak or letting them talk as you engage in another activity (checking in on Foursquare, perhaps?), one important step toward building intimacy in your relationship is by actively listening. This means that you are not just *hearing* what they have to say but *listening* to the content of their speech and responding to what they just said in kind. It seems simple, but this can help your partner feel heard, appreciated, and loved, all those good things that you *want* them to feel, but you just haven't known how to do.

Active listening can also be helpful when you're in a disagreement with your partner. Here are some tools you can use during a fight so you can get back to the fun stuff. You know, the make-up sex. Here's what to do. During a fight—or when you need to bring something to your partner's attention that you know they're not going to want to hear (especially if it's some part of them that you want them to change)—try to begin your sentences with "I feel" rather than "You." Doing so helps put your partner more at ease, or at least less on the defensive. Also, try to stay away from exaggerating words such as "always" or "never." Think about it—how would you feel if someone said to you, "You never do X" or "You always do Y"? Your immediate response is to say, "No, I don't!" instead of listening to try and understand what they're trying to convey to you.

If you're listening to your partner and keeping in mind the use of your "You" and exaggerative statements but your partner *still* doesn't feel heard, here's one more thing you can try. When they finish their thought, say something akin to "What you are saying is . . . " and then relay the message you heard to make sure that you are understanding each other.

Hopefully these tips will help you and your partner communicate easier and with greater understanding and empathy, which will all pay off later . . . in the bedroom!

67. Gaze Into Each Other's Eyes

Another important way to build intimacy is by gazing—not staring psycho killer–like—into your partner's eyes. After all, the eyes are supposedly the windows to the soul. But did you also know that when a woman that a man is attracted to looks directly into his eyes, it causes his brain to release the pleasure-causing chemical dopamine? That means if he's into you, you shouldn't be shy about holding his stare, as the result is he'll feel more connected to you. And with connection comes more oxytocin and with that, you guessed it, a better orgasm.

If you feel too vulnerable when you're looking into his eyes, or just plain weird, that's okay. But it's important to give it a try when you're with a partner that you trust or to address the underlying issues of why you feel uncomfortable with this type of intimate connection.

68. Create Romance

Romance isn't all grand gestures. It's not all walks on the beach and dinners by candlelight. It's the little things. The unexpected, thoughtful things that make your partner feel cared for. Plus, with those smaller gestures, the mood tends to be more relaxed so both of you have a chance to take the spirit of romance behind closed doors when the moment strikes. Here are a few ideas to get you started: Cook a meal for your partner after a long day at work or with the kids. Leave a love note on your partner's car. Surprise your lover with flowers and a lunch in the morning if you know he or she is going to have a busy day. Take your partner to a sporting event to see a favorite team. Grab and hold your partner's hand when you're at the dinner table. Give a big, close hug every time you see your partner. When you act selflessly and unexpectedly, your partner is likely to really appreciate it, and you'll see the payoff in the bedroom.

69. Silence, Please! Try Word Fasting

One unique way to build intimacy is through not speaking. If you're someone who finds it difficult not to talk, this exercise is especially great, as you'll have to learn to be comfortable with not filling the room with conversation. But for any couple, this exercise is a fantastic way to get to know your partner just by watching their body language. Together, pick a day (or even just a few hours) during which you two will agree to be silent. This also means you're not permitted to e-mail, text, or write notes to each other on paper.

However, looking, laughing, and definitely touching each other are all permitted. When the designated time for the completion of the word fast has been reached, discuss what the experience of being silent was like for you. Did you enjoy it? Hate it? Did either of you learn anything that you want to integrate into your relationship?

70. Be Open about Your Desires

In new relationships or in relationships where sex has become routine and dull, it can be difficult to find the words to express your sexual desires to your lover. But, while it's important to pick your battles—this is one worth picking! Your sexual happiness is important. And as most men love to please, having the confidence to tell them how they can better pleasure you is a win-win for both of you. As long as you do it with tact and aplomb and don't bark orders at the poor guy, he'll likely be enthusiastic to adjust his style. Just make sure to reward him by letting him know how good his new movements feel when he does. And who knows? Maybe he was hoping you would break the ice so you two could get out of your rut or so he could suggest something fun in the bedroom, too!

71. Use a Bead Jar

In her book *Forty Beads*, Carolyn Evans suggests that couples keep a jar next to the bed. If the man tries to make a move and the woman declines, the man puts a bead in the jar and the woman must be ready to have sex with him within the next twenty-four hours. When the deed is done, the bead is removed. Uh-huh. (For the record, putting time limits or bargaining elements on sexual activities is not fair, kind, or considerate. It puts undue pressure on your partner and can breed resentment. Besides, don't you want to engage in sex with someone who is willing and interested?)

How about this twist instead? Place a jar next to your bed and find fun objects—wine corks, keys, marbles, etc.—and every time you want to do something nice between the sheets for your partner, you put that object in the jar. This signifies to your partner that sometime within the next twenty-four hours you're going to pleasure them in any way they desire in the bedroom. The knowledge that you're going to jump their bones and give them an amazing orgasm will certainly heighten their anticipation for the moment to arrive.

72. Give Feedback

Communicating what you want in bed is one thing. Letting your partner know whether or not they're doing it right is another. While moans communicate to your partner that you're feeling pleasure, sometimes it takes a little more than nonverbal communication to fully explain your needs. After all, your partner doesn't live inside your body and can't possibly know exactly how you like to be touched unless you show or tell them. When you give feedback, be constructive. Let him know if you'd like it "a little to the left," or move him where you need him by using your hands. Or, if you're feeling dry, tell him, "I think we need more lube." Just also make sure to throw in compliments such as, "Wow, that feels incredible!" when he hits the sweet spot. By being clearer about how he's pleasuring you, you're more likely to develop a deeper sexual connection with him and you're more likely to hit the big O.

The same goes for him. If you sense that he's shy about sharing his desires and giving feedback in the bedroom, encourage him to open up by asking him to take your hand and show you how he likes to touch himself. Or as you're going down on him or manually stimulating him, pause every so often to ask him questions such as,

"Do you like it like this or would you prefer your (insert your preferred name for his male organ here) touched softer/rougher/differently?" As long as you indicate that you're interested in pleasuring him as well, he'll likely start to open up and become less shy about letting you know how he can best reach orgasm.

73. Be Honest about Your Past

No, this doesn't mean you have to confess that you mooned everyone on the highway after too many martinis at your friend's bachelorette party or that you gave your college boyfriend a blow job in the parking lot. It means that you need to be honest about your sexual history and open about any sexually transmitted infections you might have so that you and your partner can take the necessary precautions and be smart about sex. If you're thinking about having sex together, here are some questions you might want to ask to ensure your sexual escapades begin smoothly. And having peace of mind will only help you have a great orgasm.

- Do you have any STIs that you are aware of?
- When was the last time you were tested for STIs? What did they find?
- What kind of sexual activity have you had since you were last tested? Did you use protection? Were bodily fluids exchanged?

If you and your partner are not 100 percent sure whether or not you have an STI, you should make sure to use condoms to protect yourselves. That said, some STIs, such as herpes, can be transmitted even if no bodily fluids are exchanged, which is all the more reason to make sure you are both tested. If you don't have easy access to a doctor, go to your local Planned Parenthood clinic. They should be able to perform a blood test for you at a reduced cost.

DID YOU KNOW?

I don't want to alarm you, but there are estimated to be 65 million people in America living with STIs. And, for instance, did you know that 35 percent of people who have herpes don't even know it, and 75 percent of women who have chlamydia don't know it? So, be smart. Before you have sex with a new partner, make sure both of you are tested. And if it's been less than three months since one of you has had another sexual partner, be sure to use condoms until you're tested at the three-month mark, as some STIs can take time to register positive.

74. Know When to Use Protection

There are a wide variety of options to help you have safe sex. From products that cover the penis to those that surround the finger to those that drape over female genitals, there is something on the market that is designed to prevent direct contact between the sex organs and thus prevent the transmission of STIs and, in some cases, pregnancy. A condom is essentially a protective sheath that rolls down the penis and catches the ejaculatory fluid, or come. Condoms come in various materials, but latex condoms are the most durable and, when used properly, are able to protect an uninfected partner from HIV and pregnancy. If you are allergic to latex, use a polyurethane condom in its place. Female condoms that fit inside the vagina are also available, though they are still not commonly used. Dental dams are square pieces of latex that cover the female's genitals when her partner is performing oral sex. Finger cots, or condoms for a single finger, are particularly useful for anal stimulation or playing with the genitals.

75. Have Fun with Protection

When you're putting on your protective gear, make it a sensual experience in and of itself. When he's ready to be inside you, take the condom in your hands and roll it onto his penis as he's running his hands all over your naked body. Or, if he prefers to put it on, kiss, lick, and touch other parts of him to help him stay aroused. Just because you're being safe doesn't mean you have to be boring!

76. Enjoy the Afterglow

During this intimate time, you may feel very close to your partner—women's bodies release feel-good chemicals that bond them to their partner just after orgasm—and that the lovemaking has strengthened a bond between the two of you. Indulge in this sensation if it feels right instead of shying away into a less intimate space because of fear. However, if you and your partner were really just in it for a quickie, a tender kiss and a few sweet words should suffice.

And if you're looking for another romp, that's great—just keep in mind that at first you need to be gentle with your partner's genitals. Following an orgasm, the clitoris and penis are very sensitive, and your partner may even shy away from your touch. After a certain period of time (which depends on your partner), your partner might be ready to go again, but you need to be patient. While you're waiting, touch and kiss your partner's other erogenous zones to try to rebuild sexual arousal.

77. Heal the Fear of Intimacy

As you create intimacy within your romantic life with the help of the tips I've suggested, keep in mind that some people have a fear of intimacy. This fear may stem from a history of being rejected, betrayed, or abandoned in nonromantic or romantic relationships. Or it could result from them being inexperienced in the bedroom, feeling less than confident about their body image, or having a fear of losing their identity within the relationship. Depending on your partner's history, certain events may trigger the fear of intimacy within him. For instance, you may find that although you know he cares for you, he pulls away during the afterglow or that he has a difficult time holding your gaze.

If you begin to see signs of this fear and if this relationship is important to you, you may want to consider couple's counseling or suggest your partner seek counseling on their own to work through their issues so you two can build a healthy romantic life together. If their fear of intimacy is relatively mild, letting them know and showing them that you can be trusted should help assuage their fear over time.

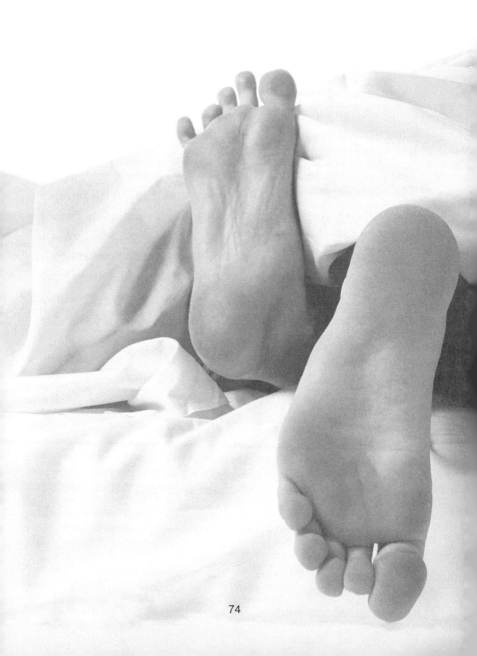

CHAPTER FIVE

Pleasure Yourself First

78. Pleasure Yourself

Now begins the fun stuff that you've been waiting for. You've found ways to become comfortable with your body, you've set the scene, you've learned how to relax, and you're now ready to have a great orgasm.

One way to begin is by getting in touch with yourself. Literally. Growing up you probably heard all of the reasons why you shouldn't masturbate: you'll go blind, you'll get hairy palms, it's dirty, blah, blah, blah. I could go on. But masturbation is the best way to learn what works for you sexually (as well as what doesn't), and learning about your sexual self will make you that much more confident and capable in the bedroom. Plus, masturbation can:

- Relieve headaches and stress
- Keep the pelvic floor toned, preventing urinary incontinence in older people
- Give you a break from sexual tension
- Alleviate menstrual cramps

Masturbation is also the safest form of sexual pleasure you can enjoy. So before you jump into bed with someone else, jump in bed with yourself. You'll be glad you did.

79. Take Your Time and Disregard Distractions

Masturbation isn't something that should be rushed. Of course, there are times when we're feeling stimulated and just want to get off quickly and be done with it so we can get back to focusing on another activity; but when you're exploring your body and finding out what arouses you, you don't want to feel rushed. For these solo sessions, set aside some time for yourself when you won't be under stress to go somewhere or have a looming to-do list.

Also, turn off your cell phone. This will not only squash your urge to check what those in your social network are up to, it will also prevent anyone from texting or calling you when you're almost there.

80. Tap Into Your Imagination

For most of us, desire starts with a single thought or visual cue. When you're on your own, even before you start touching yourself, start thinking about those things that turn you on. Refer back to that arousal map you created in Tip 44 and take yourself through your list of answers. If you love the feel of warm water on your skin, head off to the shower or bath. If you love a certain scent, light a candle. If there's a certain person or celebrity you're attracted to, imagine that person lying on your bed or walking through the door. Fantasize about how that might play out. Use the knowledge you took the time to explore earlier to turn yourself on when you're on your own.

81. Have Fun with Visual Stimulation

While some people are able to rely mostly on their imagination to become aroused when masturbating, some require more direct visual stimulation to reach orgasm. That is just one of the reasons that men in particular enjoy porn (their brains are evolutionarily hard-wired for easy arousal and it's almost just as easy for them to be stimulated by an image as it is by action). But, though most porn has been developed for the male viewer, that doesn't mean that there aren't images you can use to stimulate yourself visually. If traditional pornography—images or videos—aren't your cup of tea, then consider watching a video designed specifically for female viewers. These movies often feature real-life couples engaged in more sensual acts. Or, find an image of someone you think is attractive. Look at it and let your imagination go wild while you're pleasuring yourself.

FUN FACT

For a moment, I'm going to sound like the mother you never had. Porn is fine, but too much of it—like too much of anything, frankly—can be detrimental to your sex life. Recently, scientists discovered that continual overstimulation of the libido has the power to desensitize your dopamine production. Dopamine is the body's primary "desire" chemical, so if its release only happens when triggered by over-sexualized imagery, you can imagine how this could be a problem. So, enjoy your porn . . . just in moderation.

82. Try a Different Position

How do you usually masturbate? While sitting? Standing? Lying on your back? Against the wall of the shower? Just because you're on your own doesn't give you a free pass to be lazy (although sometimes it's okay if you are). It's time to try something new. Experiment with a position you haven't tried before. Twist your legs together for a different type of sensation. Try using your other hand. Because while you might find that, no, you can't come on your hands and knees, you also might discover a better position in which to stimulate yourself than the one you've been relying on for years. And possibly a better orgasm as well!

83. Change Locations

It's important to be comfortable while you're masturbating, especially if you've never had an orgasm before or often have a difficult time reaching climax. But once you've gotten more effective at masturbating to orgasm, feel free to move around! If you're feeling bored in your bedroom, try out different locations in your home like the shower, the bath, or the top of the dryer, and even consider going outside into nature. The thrill of changing places, and possibly getting caught, may give you an even bigger rush.

84. Make Noise!

When you pleasure yourself, don't be shy. Instead of holding all those good feelings in, let them out! It might feel ridiculous at first, but letting go and moaning or saying whatever comes to mind can be a total turn-on. It also will likely help you to have an even better orgasm because you're not focused on holding anything back. Making noise also helps you release your breath, which you might have not even noticed you were holding! If others are in the house, turn on some music to drown out your moans before you get going.

85. Touch Yourself Indirectly

You may think of masturbating as just a means to an end, but you don't always have to take the fast track and enjoy no-frills masturbating. Every so often, don't touch your genitals immediately. Try stimulating some of your erogenous zones. Run your fingers through your hair to stimulate your scalp, trace the curve of your stomach, run your nails along your thighs . . . find what works for you. And if you're worried you might be silly, just ask yourself: Who is watching? No one has to know what you do alone in the privacy of your own bedroom if you don't want to tell them. As you engage in self-love—not only of the genitals but the whole body—you'll feel those fires burning even brighter down below.

86. Touch Yourself Directly

By now, after some time spent stimulating the rest of your body, you've likely worked yourself up into quite an aroused state. This is the best time to place your hands right on your genitals. Place your hand on top of your vulva (this is the entire vaginal area) and start to move it around slowly. Find and stimulate your clitoris. Pull on and play with your labia. Try inserting one finger into your vagina. Find the sensations that feel good and continue those. Then, go on a search to find others. Don't be afraid to experiment with varying degrees of pressure in your quest to discover what turns you on the most. Even if it's something you've never considered, trust yourself and your body and make the leap. You may find you love it.

87. Tease Yourself for a Bigger O!

A great way to suddenly increase your sexual pleasure and desire when you're masturbating is by teasing yourself. When you are close to reaching orgasm—or if you're having trouble getting past the plateau stage—take one hand off of your vagina and place it somewhere else you find erogenous. As you stimulate your erogenous zones with one hand, use the other to go close, but not touch your vulva. Pinch, scratch, use finger-light touches, and even consider licking your body for the purpose of arousal. By building sexual tension, you'll be able to heighten the release that you're looking for. Then, return both hands to your vulva and bring yourself to what will likely be a very powerful climax.

88. Go Hands-Free

Everyone's doing it. Well, maybe not in bed, but in many other places in their lives. It's an age of voice-activated chat, Bluetooth headsets, remote keys to unlock cars, and so on. If you've never considered trying to masturbate without using your hands, it's worth at least a try. Set aside more time than usual to pleasure yourself, and then spark your desire and excitement visually or with your imagination. Imagine you or your ideal sexual partner touching you until you get worked up to the point of orgasm or until you just can't help but reach out and touch yourself. If you can't manage to come without using your hands, that's okay, as few people can, but it's just one more step to getting to know yourself even better.

89. Get Wet with Lubricant

Why should you go out and buy lubricant when plain old saliva has done the trick for years? Because saliva, while useful, dries quickly. If you have trouble staying wet while masturbating—or during sex—lubricants can help keep your genitals continually wet so you can enjoy pleasuring yourself for a longer period of time without the need to reapply. Lubricants can also help reduce friction in the vagina or anus and on the penis during sexual play when your natural lubrication isn't enough. With friction comes chafing and pain, and the last thing you want to do when trying to pleasure yourself is to make yourself physically uncomfortable. That said, women should avoid using creams, lotions, or anything scented near the vagina, as these can irritate it and trigger yeast infections.

90. Try Water-Based Lubricants

Water-based lubricants are the most popular and the most recommended type of lubricants. They have been developed to be nonstaining, nonirritating, and safe to use with all condoms and sex toys. With the exception of those flavored for oral sex, most are tasteless and all are easy to wash off from yourself, your sheets, your toys, and your partner with soap and water. They're not your only option, but they are a good starting place. They come in two main consistencies: liquid and jelly. The liquid types resemble a slicker version of your saliva and natural fluids, while the jelly types are noticeably thicker but last longer. If you are preparing for anal play or an extended sexual romp, opt for the jelly kind. But either way, these water-based lubricants can help keep the fun going for longer and increase your chances of experiencing an amazing orgasm.

91. Experiment with Oil as Lubricant

Another type of lubricant you could use while masturbating or during sex are plant-based oils, which feel great on the skin. If you've ever thumbed through a beauty magazine, you've probably come across an article touting the wonderful effects of safflower oil, olive oil, or avocado oil. Their high fat content makes them excellent moisturizers, so even if you don't end up using them in the bedroom, try integrating them into your grooming routine.

But back to erotic play. The primary problem with oils is that they can weaken latex, so they shouldn't be used with any latex condoms or sex toys. If you are using other methods of birth control—or are using vinyl condoms—then give your favorite natural vegetable oil a try. One fun one is coconut. It smells incredible and is easier to wash out of sheets, hair, etc. than other types. However, don't use synthetic oil-based lubricants, such as petroleum jelly. These not only break down latex, they also tend to remain in the vagina or anus, which is uncomfortable and can lead to infection.

92. Slip and Slide with Silicone-Based Lubricants

Silicone-based lubricants are the slipperiest and longest-lasting lubricants on the market that are made for personal, sexual use. And when we're talking about sex, *slippery* and *long-lasting* are good words to consider. If you're planning on doing it in the water without a condom, use these since they won't rinse off. However, be careful if you're using them indoors, as you don't want to crack your skull by slipping on a droplet. Also, these aren't the ideal lubricants to use with condoms or silicone-based toys. They can cause condoms to break and they can degrade the materials in the sex toy, making it dangerous and unusable. For condoms and toys, use a water-based lubricant. But if you're actually in the water, think of Baywatch and opt for silicone.

93. Stimulate Your Vulva

A woman's primary sex organ is the vulva, which consists of the inner and outer labia, the clitoris, and the vaginal opening. So let's talk about how to touch it in a way that will help you achieve orgasm. You may find it easy to turn yourself on by using some or all of the techniques I've mentioned, or it may take a few tries before you finally feel a spark. Either way, just go at your own pace. Before you move directly to touching the vulva, spend time running your hands over your other erogenous zones until you're starting to feel good and are ready to move forward. When you do so, you may need a little extra lubrication or your own saliva, or natural fluids may be enough. Just don't go in dry. It'll be painful. Now is not the time or place to push forward in the face of adversity. Applying lubrication can be a sensual act in itself. Use gentle strokes across your vagina's opening, up either side of the opening, and then end with your finger on your clitoris. Repeat this as long as it feels pleasurable, pausing between each stroke to allow yourself a moment to get excited in anticipation. Now start to explore the various areas of the vulva, allowing yourself to be guided by what you find pleasurable. Experiment with the direction and pressure of the strokes, and try gently squeezing or pinching the labia or clitoris.

94. Pay Special Attention to the Clitoris

As you learn what feels good for you down below, you'll probably notice that your clitoris is your hot button of sexual excitement. However, you may find that touching it directly is too intense a sensation for you and that touching it through its clitoral hood is more pleasurable. Every woman's body is different, so it's up to you to experiment. Here are some ways to stimulate it if you do find touching it indirectly or directly to be exhilarating. Try taking your clitoris and pinching it between two fingers and gliding the hood back and forth over it. Try stroking it from side to side using varying degrees of pressure. Then try circles or figure eights.

95. Experiment with the Clock Exercise

While you've been playing around with your clitoris, you may have noticed that one side is more sensitive than another. It may be surprising, but even though the glans of the clitoris is small (at least when compared with the corresponding male glans), the nerve endings are not evenly distributed across it. Some reports say the upper left quadrant is the most sensitive and responsive to pleasure. But other studies suggest that the ten o'clock and two o'clock positions (think of this clock as if you are facing the clitoris, not looking down on it from above) are the most sensitive. Try touching yourself in all of these areas to discover which one makes you squirm in delight and inch closer to orgasm more than the others.

96. Love Your Vagina

Though some women can climax through clitoral stimulation alone, others need penetration. This can be accomplished just by using sex toys or your hands. While playing with your vulva, and adding some lubrication if necessary, tease yourself a bit by pushing your middle finger just a little way into your vagina and trying to keep your palm on top of your clitoris. This allows you to simultaneously stimulate the most sensitive part of your vagina and your clitoris. As you start feeling more turned on, you might want to lie on your stomach to give your clitoris and pubic bone a little extra pressure as they push against your hand. Use gentle rocking motions, moving up and down on your finger—and adding another if it seems like it would feel good—until you bring yourself to a mind-blowing climax.

97. Try a Blended Orgasm

Now that you've been experimenting with various ways to pleasure yourself, it's time for you to try a more advanced technique: The Blended Orgasm. This is an orgasm that involves both the clitoris and the G-spot. Here's how to reach it: When you are fully turned on and are able to easily slide your finger in and out of your vagina, reach in and try to locate your G-spot. It is a small but ridged and slightly raised area on the front wall of your vagina. And now that you've touched it, you may feel like you have to pee. Hold that thought. Though this is a feeling you're not accustomed to, stimulating this area won't cause you to urinate all over your sheets. Just continue to play with it and those signals will transform into an intense feeling of arousal that will bring you to the brink of being ready to come. At the same time, put your thumb or finger from the other hand on your clitoris and stimulate it in a way that you enjoy. Cue amazing orgasm.

98. Try the Showerhead

The shower can be a great masturbatory aid. One way you can take advantage of this mundane bathroom fixture is to position yourself so that the water is falling directly onto your clitoris. Touch your vulva and other erogenous zones at the same time and you'll be excited in no time. If you have a removable showerhead, you can put it against your vulva to experience a steady or pulsating stream of water.

99. Touch Your Perineum

I've mentioned the perineum before as one of the primary erogenous zones, but I want to give you a few tips on how to stimulate it. While you're masturbating, take one or two fingers of your other hand and press on this space. Begin gently and then work up the pressure as there are many nerves here, but the added pressure may cause added pleasure and result in a more intense orgasm.

100. Stimulate Your Anus

For the most part, you've probably focused on your primary sex organs while you're masturbating. But it's important to branch out from time to time. One of the ways you can do this is by playing with your butt. While you're touching your vulva with one hand, reach around and play with your booty with the other. Caress it, slap it, knead it, whatever you like. After some time doing this, start by rubbing your finger on your anus in slow circles (you may need a little lubrication), and when you're ready, slowly slip a finger inside. Move it around gently inside to see how it feels if you've never done this before. You may find that you have an orgasm out of nowhere. Later on, if you want to go back to using two hands on your vagina after you've engaged in anal play, just remember to wash your hands first.

101. For Him: Stimulate Your Penis

Though I have an inkling that if you're reading this book, you're female, it is possible that I am mistaken. To that end, I want to provide my male readers with some masturbatory guidance to supplement their existing knowledge on the subject. As you know, a man's primary sex organ is the penis. And while you may have been masturbating since your early teenage years, I've got a few tips and tricks that may help to increase your pleasure. Begin by placing some saliva (or, ideally, a water-based lubricant) on the tips of your middle and index fingers and on the thumb of the hand you want to use. Start by gently stroking the head of the penis down to the base. Then, when you reach the bottom, place your hand on top of the glans and start again. Continue doing this, varying the pressure, until you're ready for another type of stimulation. Add more lubrication and this time, instead of using just your fingers and thumb, use your entire hand. Continue to stroke your penis with a downward motion, lifting your hand each time you reach the base. Even though this feels great, don't rush. Pause between each stroke of the shaft and head. Breathe. Anticipate the next wave of pleasure. This will let the sensation build slowly and allow you to focus more on the pleasure before it ends with a powerful ejaculation.

102. For Him: Play with Your Testicles

While you're stimulating your penis and getting more and more aroused, try taking the other hand and using it to fondle your testicles. Start by running your fingers gently over your scrotum. Then, slowly begin to massage each testicle.

Try cupping them and moving your hand from the back to the front to stimulate all of the areas that you've overlooked in previous one-on-one sessions. Find the areas that give you goose bumps or a pleasurable shudder and continue to pay attention to those. Another way to stimulate the testicles is by pulling gently on the scrotum. Some guys enjoy tugging on it quite hard. But since—as I'm sure you know—this is a very sensitive area, begin with a light touch and work your way up to rougher play, as in this case, unexpected pain will undoubtedly lead to a delayed orgasm.

103. For Him: Use the Other Hand

For women, attempting to use the other hand during masturbation is an exercise in futility and frustration. More often than not, it results in fumbled attempts at pleasure and an inability to get the right angle to properly stimulate the right spots. It also gives us a deeper appreciation for your ability to bring us to orgasm with only your hands. But for men, masturbating while using the other hand isn't as complicated. And because of that, switching to the other hand can give you the sensation of being touched by someone else. The result? Possibly, a more intense orgasm.

104. For Him: Use the Shower

A few steps back, I told women how to use the shower as a mastur-batory aid. But men can take advantage of the shower as well. Align yourself so that the steady stream of the shower—or, preferably, the faucet of the bathtub—falls onto the glans of your penis. Focus on this sensation as you begin to stroke your shaft and pleasure your-self. Tease yourself by moving the glans in and out of the stream until you bring yourself to orgasm. If you have a removable show-erhead, try this more intense move: Lie on the floor of the shower, put your penis underneath you so that it faces your feet (I know this move is a little unconventional. Try it anyway.), and hold the show-erhead in such a way that you can alternate between stimulating the shaft and the glans. The combination of the pressure and the water stimulation should result in a great orgasm.

105. For Him: Master Ejaculation

If you've been having a difficult time during sexual play because of your tendency to ejaculate prematurely, use masturbation as a tool to slow yourself down. When you're starting to approach orgasm, pay attention to the sensations that you are feeling. Do you feel a sensation of movement in your genitals? Does your breath quicken? Do you have the sensation that you must come . . . *now*?

By being aware of your body's involuntary responses to pleasure and recognizing the point of no return, you can train yourself to stop coming before you want the event to be over.

Practice this for a few solo sessions, and then, once you believe you've found the point at which you can stop yourself and pull back from ejaculating, and the point at which you can't, try this exercise: When you're close to coming, but not yet at that unstoppable point, stop masturbating for a moment and distract yourself by thinking of things other than those that would turn you on. If you still feel like you're ready to explode, place your thumb and index finger around the base of your penis or below the glans (try one method for one "rep" and the other method for another to see which method works best for you) and squeeze for twenty to thirty seconds. Once you no longer feel the immediate need to come, begin to get yourself close to orgasm again and stop yourself using the aforementioned method. Repeat this exercise several times before you finally let yourself ejaculate. Your orgasm should be incredibly powerful.

One more trick to help you with coming prematurely is to try squeezing your PC muscle just before that "point of no return." For ʼting your PC muscle, see Tips 253–256.

Him: Try an Artificial Vagina

:o play with dildos and vibrators, I think men should ht to use artificial sex organs to stimulate themselves if they so choose. Artificial vaginas (also known as "pocket pussies") come in a wide range of styles, from those that are cast straight from the vaginas of adult porn stars to those that look like a mouth that you can slide into to simulate oral sex. Other artificial vaginas are a little more discreet, some resembling lotion bottles or just a plain silicone sheath you might put over a sword—in this case your own. With any of these, lubrication is necessary, so I've taken particular notice of the Tenga toys, prelubricated toys that are filled on the inside with ridges, like a real vagina, and even use a bit of suction to help you achieve a great orgasm. Want to try one out but feel too shy to walk into a sex store and buy one? That, my friend, is what the Internet was made for. Well, that and cat videos.

107. For Him: Try a Sex Doll

If you've been enjoying your pocket pussy but want to take it a step farther, there is one step beyond this: The sex doll. Unless you've seen *Lars and the Real Girl*, your idea of a sex doll may resemble those inflatable dolls that used to be commonplace at bachelor parties. They're not necessarily a bad option, but I can't imagine that their hard seams and super-slick plastic are terribly fun to have sex with. They are, however, much less expensive than the realistic sex dolls on the market. But there's a reason. Those sex dolls look and feel (mostly) like touching and having sex with a real person. Each doll will run you a couple thousand dollars—but they're durable and receive mostly rave reviews from their customers. However, if you are in a relationship, sit down and discuss the idea that you want to order a sex doll with your partner, as this may not sit well with her. During this conversation, you can address her concerns as well as your reasoning for wanting a sex doll. If your reasons are tied to your dissatisfaction with your current sexual relationship, this could also be the time to begin to work through those issues (i.e., before spending thousands on an inanimate object).

DID YOU KNOW?

If you want to have great sex and experience intimacy, a willingness to be sexually vulnerable is a must. Most people protect themselves when they are around other people. This is true even in sex. We tend to be wary of others hurting us, so we keep a layer of protection around our hearts just in case. Then, if a partner does something that we associate with rejection, criticism, or any of our other favorite fears, we say, "I knew it! I knew this would happen! It's a good thing I didn't let myself get completely vulnerable—because then, I'd be even more hurt."

Opening up to your partner is an act of great trust. It is the most important thing you can do for yourself if you want to heal your old wounds and realize that you can trust yourself to deal with whatever happens to you.

Being openly vulnerable can also help you see that the pain another person's behavior triggers in you tells you that you still need to heal in yourself. Pain is not necessarily bad; it can reveal to you the areas in your unconscious belief structure that need to be updated. It shows you where you need to focus in your journey toward wholeness.

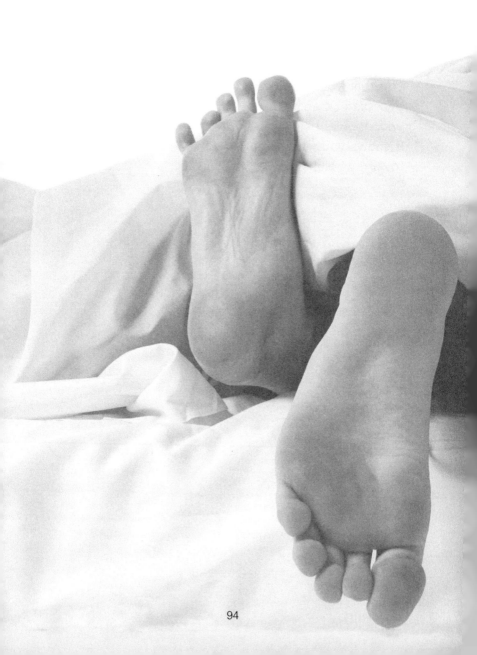

CHAPTER SIX

Create Intimacy

108. Keep Your Clothes On

Before the clothes are ripped off, the condoms are opened, and you and your lover are lying clasped in each other's arms, there are a few steps that come first: building desire, finding ways to create intimacy, and engaging in foreplay. All of those steps are necessary to set the scene for a passionate orgasm. In the tips that follow, you'll learn how to do this effectively so that by the time the clothes *do* come off, you'll both be ready for action. But first, it all begins with a little seduction.

109. Master the Art of Flirtation

Once you've found someone that has captured your attention, one of you is likely to begin trying to seduce the other by flirting, which is essentially the human version of the mating dance. Some of you may be the type who flirts without even realizing they're doing so—that's because when you flirt, you flirt with your whole body. Flirting well also requires a certain degree of confidence, as the way you dress, the way you make eye contact, how you talk, and your body language all contribute to your flirting ability. That said, the most forward advances of flirtation are made through eye contact, flirtatious talk, and body language.

DID YOU KNOW . . .

Red is not only a sexy color, it's the color that men are most attracted to. Recent research at the University of Rochester revealed that men were significantly more attracted to women who were wearing red and more likely to ask them out on an extravagant date. So, the next time you're going on a first date, or you want to turn on your mate, wear red!

110. Establish Eye Contact

When you flirt with your eyes, you do a little more than just look at someone. For women, eye flirting is a balance between showing someone you're interested by looking directly at them to catch their attention and playing a little hard to get by looking away coyly when you catch them returning your glance. The next time you're sitting at a bar or you're browsing in a store and see someone cute, try this. Look at them until you catch their attention, and then look away. Do it again a minute or two later, but this time, look toward another object of your interest (your drink, the item you're holding, etc.) and then smile shyly in that direction. Let another minute or two pass, and look at the guy again. This time, smile at him and hold his glance for a moment. Then, continue doing whatever you were doing before. He should get the hint that you're interested. If he doesn't come over, he is either shy or uninterested. But, even if he isn't interested, that's okay. After all, a little practice never hurt anyone.

111. Talk Flirtatiously

After you've established eye contact with the object of your desire, the most common next step is to strike up a conversation with them, and this is likely to involve at least some playful—or flirtatious —talk. Flirtatious talk is upbeat, fun, and sexy. As the two of you banter back and forth, playfully teasing each other and laughing at each other's jokes, you develop a rapport that may lead to the next step. Flirtatious talk—and eye flirting—aren't just for new couples or interested people who just met. They're for established couples, too! Inject a little fun back into your love life by flirting with your partner to encourage a greater sense of play in your relationship that may lead all the way back to the bedroom!

112. Move Flirtatiously

Near the beginning of the book I discussed how important it is to have confidence. Flirting is one of those key moments when having a strong sense of self and a healthy amount of self-confidence is important, and when it comes to flirting with your body—and touching another's—portraying a strong sense of self-confidence shows the person you're flirting with that you have value.

Some ways you can flirt by touching yourself include playing with your hair with your fingers, uncrossing and crossing your legs slowly (but in a ladylike, not *Basic Instinct*, fashion), or doing things that call attention to your mouth or neck such as licking or biting your lips, or nonchalantly opening an article of clothing to expose bare skin. You can also flirt by touching the other person in subtle ways. Touch their leg, arm, shoulder, or back as you're talking or joking with them. Make your touches light and don't linger, as you want to convey interest and leave them wanting for more.

113. Dress Up to Arouse

Whether you're heading out on your first date or you've been married to the same partner for the last thirty years, it's important to take the time to dress up when you want to show the other person you're interested. This doesn't necessarily mean putting on a leather miniskirt or the most plunging, cleavage-baring top you own, though that may have a very positive effect on your partner. When you're dressing flirtatiously, you're likely to accentuate certain features of yourself you're most proud of. If you have toned arms you want to show off, wear a sleeveless top. If you want to show off your legs, wear a skirt of reasonable length with a slit in it so the man gets the pleasure of the peek-a-boo factor every once in a while. You could also draw attention to the areas you want to highlight with a piece of jewelry or another accessory, such as a watch or scarf, or just by wearing a fabric that begs to be touched.

FUN FACT

Your cycle not only affects your mood and how much you're craving certain foods (pass the burger, please). It also affects the way you dress. Near the time you're ovulating, you're more likely to dress sexier in the hopes of attracting a mate while you're super fertile.

114. Wear Tantalizing Perfume

Earlier in this book, I mentioned how filling your home with certain scents can turn your partner on. The same goes for perfume. While men love the smell of lavender, vanilla, and pumpkin pie, women prefer more musky odors like licorice. Keep this in mind when picking out what you'll be dabbing on later. Just make sure to err on the light side. A little whiff is sexy; causing your lover to wonder if you bathed in the stuff, not so much. These aren't Elizabethan times, after all!

115. Wear Sexy Underwear Every Day

If you've watched *Mad Men*, then you know that back in the 1940s and 1950s, women wore sexy undergarments underneath their clothes. The bras and panties of the day accentuated their curves, and it likely gave them the same confident, knowing feeling you get today when you wear hot underwear under an everyday outfit. Just having the secret knowledge that you're wearing something seductive when you're at the office or running errands about town can turn you on! And, when you take off your clothes and your partner gets to see the lingerie or underwear you've got on, you're sure to raise eyebrows in the best way possible. There are all types of sexy lingerie out there that you can wear depending on what mood you want to inspire, but here's a rundown of the basics.

- Demi Bra—The bra is intended to hold up the breasts. These also have a double purpose as they prop up the breasts but reveal the nipples or allow very easy access to them.
- Teddy—These one-piece garments are often made from lace, cotton, satin, or silk and are essentially the nightgown's sexier sister. They come in a variety of styles, some which allow the breasts to show.
- Corset—If you want something that will make your breasts perkier and your waist smaller, step away from the shapers and toward the classic corset. Whether the corset you choose laces or fastens up the back, it's hard to think of anything sexier. Just try not to wear it when you might be doing a lot of sitting. While modern corsets are significantly more comfortable than those of the Victorian era (thanks primarily to the fact that the boning in them is made from flexible plastic instead of whale bones), they're still not the easiest to sit in for long periods of time.
- Garter Belt—This lacy piece of lingerie fastens around your waist and is intended to hold up a pair of thigh-high stockings or fishnets.

116. For Him: Send Lingerie to Your Lover

This one is for my male readers: The movies can be a great source of inspiration for ideas—even if some of them are a little far-fetched. This is one of those. It's worth trying, even if you only ever try it once. With your lover's size in mind, head to your nearest lingerie store or high-end boutique and select an outfit that you know your partner would love and that you find tantalizing. Have the sales clerk wrap it prettily and then have this delivered to your lover's office with a mysterious note along the lines of "I'd love to see you in this tonight." Just try to be as discreet as possible about it so it doesn't attract the attention of nosy coworkers.

For my female readers, when you pick up some new, sexy lingerie and want to wear it for your beau, take advantage of the use of your smartphone. Snap a photo of just part of the item and send it to his phone. His mind will start racing with anticipation to see what the rest of it looks like . . . and what it looks like on you. Before it falls to the floor, of course.

117. Go Commando

If you're the type of woman who always wears underwear, that's great. Keeping your lady parts dry, clean, and covered will cut down on potential yeast infections. But, one night, when you know you'll be meeting with your partner and that a rendezvous is likely, try going sans blooms. One way to get things moving in a sexy direction is to wear a dress or a skirt and, at some point during the night, lean over and let your partner know you're not wearing any panties. If that doesn't turn him on, check him for a pulse.

118. Try Shaving . . . or Not

What's attractive "down there" has changed dramatically over the years. In the '70s, a full bush ruled. In the '90s, the fully shaven look or landing strip took over. And these days, it seems anything goes. To mix things up a bit, try a new look. If you usually go *au natural,* tidy up your look or consider going bare. He might show his appreciation for the gesture with more enthusiasm for oral sex, as it will be easier for him to give you pleasure when he's not having to remove hairs from his mouth during the act. If you usually are bare or rock very little pubic hair, try growing it all—or at least some—out. One of the drawbacks to shaving the pubic hair is that the hairs catch pheromones—chemicals that attract you to your partner—and the movement of those hair follicles may help you reach orgasm, so you may find your orgasms are better with more going on down there!

119. Build Sexual Tension

Do you ever feel the heat between you and another person? That feeling that builds until you feel like you're ready to explode with lust and jump the bones of the person you're feeling the spark with? That's sexual tension. At times, it feels like it comes out of the blue. The two of you are just sitting there when suddenly, something sparks it until it becomes a raging inferno. Other times, it takes a lot of effort to generate. But the effort is worth it, as often, when sexual tension is highest, the orgasm can be more powerful. To create sexual tension between you and your partner you need two things: safety and danger or excitement. If your sex life has been a little too serious lately, try injecting a bit of fun and play into it. Do something unexpected— outside the bedroom—that takes the pressure off and you may find that leads to more passion between the sheets.

120. Get Dirty on the Dance Floor

Dancing is excellent exercise but it's also a great way to get you closer to an incredible orgasm. That's because it helps put you more in touch with your body in a way that allows you to release your inhibitions and get into the groove. It also allows you to show off your personality through the movements you make when you're lighting up the dance floor. Are you an extrovert who really gets into the beat or do you prefer to just move a little bit? As you're dancing, you might find someone whose dance style is compatible with yours and the sparks could fly!

Dancing with this new person, or with your partner, in a suggestive way hints to your dance partner that you want more than just a little spin around the floor. Dancing in this manner may include a lot of bumping and grinding or booty shaking of the pelvic area. Often your whole body ends up touching and moving with that of your dance partner. Sometimes it even ends with the woman rubbing against the man's leg and the man getting an erection. Who knows—you might have to pop into a dark corner to do something about this sudden "problem". That said, there are other, more traditional types of suggestive dances, like the tango, that aren't so overtly sexual but through which sexual tension is built up throughout the dance. By the end of the number, you'll definitely be able to feel the sexual fire burning between the two of you.

121. Watch a Burlesque Show or Striptease Together

Burlesque stars would be aghast if they found out I lumped them in with strippers, but for our purposes, the two performances have similar effects on getting you both into the bedroom. In both routines, there's some stripping of clothing involved and acts that may replicate those you've done in the bedroom. Burlesque is more about the tease, the costuming, and the artful performance, which can range from humorous to sensual. While at a strip club, there isn't nearly as much mystery. It's more about being visually tantalized by the naked—or nearly naked—bodies of the dancers. That said, in both, men or women are using sexually suggestive, or just plain sexual, moves to entice their audience. Before you surprise your partner with a trip to the burlesque or strip club, make sure that this is something your partner is comfortable with and go over what is acceptable behavior and what is not before you arrive. Some men or women might get aroused by the sight of a stripper giving their partner a lap dance, while others will just feel turned off. It's best to know where your partner's limits lie before you cross that line. (This goes double for you—if something is not okay with you, don't say that it is.)

122. Flip on a Porno

If you (or your partner) don't feel entirely comfortable with the idea of a strip club, than a potentially safer route is looking at porn within the privacy of your own home. One way to do this is to sit down with your lover and thumb through your favorite pornography magazine together or bring over the computer and share some of your favorite sites, images, or clips with one another. When you play together online, you might find out more about what your partner likes. Try your best not to judge, as for some, sharing the pornography they watch with their partner can cause some trepidation. But, if you're open-minded, this could turn into a fun exercise, as one of you might suggest to Google something and the pair of you could have fun exploring each other's kinkier sides as you go down the rabbit hole. Another option is to go to the adult video store together and rent or buy a film that you both would enjoy. There are countless pornography niches, and there is bound to be something to fulfill nearly every fetish or mood, whether you two want to watch real couples taping their sensual love together or feast your eyes on intense scenes of BDSM (bondage, domination, sadism, masochism) and beyond.

As you watch, the two of you might get some ideas of what you could try in the bedroom—and probably find some things that are just absurd to smirk at together—but you probably won't end up watching or flipping through images for very long before you're both eager to get it on yourselves!

123. Read Erotica to Each Other

A picture may be worth a thousand words, but for some women, pornography is a turn-off. Even if that's not the case, while men are particularly visual creatures when it comes to what arouses them, women can easily be turned on by reading about erotic scenes and picturing them in their minds. Why else do you think romance novels are so popular? It's certainly not for the Pulitzer-quality writing or gripping plot lines of most dime-store paperbacks. A great way to find out what turns on your partner is to ask your partner to read their favorite erotic scene out loud to you. Listen carefully and, if you think they might be up for it, suggest you stop reading and try out that scenario with a little role-playing. You might get so swept away in the fantasy of it that you have an orgasm for the books! In addition to pulp romance novels, there are many well-written erotic books, such as D. H. Lawrence's *Lady Chatterley's Lover*, the erotic works of Anaïs Nin, and, for those into restraint play, *The Story of O*.

124. Talk Dirty in Bed . . . or Anywhere Else!

One of the great things about watching porn and reading erotica is that it helps you develop a sexual language that has a bit more edge to it than the words I'm using in this book. When you want to turn on your partner, those are exactly the kinds of words you want to whisper in his ear. Though you might feel a little silly at first using raunchy, aggressive terminology, try telling your lover what you'd like him to do to you or ask him what he wants you to do to him. Play around with different words for each other's sex organs to see which light up your lover's eyes. Some may make both of you laugh, but there are likely a few that will perk up their ears in delight. If you want to take things a step further, keep talking dirty as you touch each other, as the heat of those words could add to the intensity of your orgasm.

125. Take It All Off, Baby

Watching someone take their clothes off seductively is hot. Even if your lover isn't into porn or strip clubs or anything of that nature, we doubt your partner will look anything but pleased if you decide to do a personalized striptease. Though the spontaneous striptease is definitely fun, you can prepare to perform one by dressing in carefully planned layers and including accessories like a hat, gloves, belt, or scarf in order to prolong the experience, as the concept is to expose just a little more skin with each removal. Start by playing some music that you think would appeal to your partner—I'd recommend slow and sensual tunes if you want to perform a seductive dance or faster, more aggressive songs if you're planning on going the dominatrix route. Ask them to sit on the bed and close their eyes until you're ready to begin. The anticipation will heighten the impact of seeing you fully dressed in your costume. When you're ready, start by slowly removing articles of clothing one at a time and find a sexy way to play with many of them before tossing them across the room, to your partner, or onto the floor. By the end of the striptease, he'll be so hot for you that it'll be hard to deny the next step is him taking you to new levels of pleasure in appreciation.

126. Give Your Partner a Lap Dance

An excellent way to end a striptease is by giving your partner a lap dance and teasing your partner by seductively rubbing your sexy body over him. Begin by asking your partner to place his hands at the sides, and let him know that under no circumstances, no matter how turned on he gets, is he allowed to touch you. Only you can do the touching. This rule helps to build great sexual tension. Start by dancing in front of your lover; come into close contact but don't touch him quite yet. When you feel he is sufficiently turned on, start brushing up against him with your naked, or nearly naked, body. Tease him by going close to his genitals and then backing away again. Then try straddling him, continuing to tease and gyrate against your lover's clothed (or, perhaps at this point, naked) penis. It may take a few songs to get your lover sufficiently hot and bothered, but soon enough your lover will be unable to resist and will have to ravish you with his love.

127. Try Aphrodisiacs

Ever heard that the way to a man's heart is through his stomach? It's always a pleasure when someone takes the time to cook for us, but there are certain foods that have been rumored to increase desire. Some of these foods include:

- Chocolate
- Avocado
- Asparagus
- Kelp
- Mangoes
- Eggs
- Kava kava
- Oysters
- Pumpkin
- Tomato
- Basil
- Tangerine
- Almonds
- Bananas
- Figs
- Maca
- Damiana
- Ginseng
- Cayenne
- Cloves
- Vanilla

Though some, such as the oyster, may have gotten their naughty reputation because they resemble female genitalia, it's still a fun process to engage in eating these foods with your lover and seeing what happens. Just stay away from any that are clearly bad for the environment, like powdered rhinoceros horn. Not so sexy!

128. Carry on a Long-Distance Relationship

If you're involved in a long-distance relationship, one where you don't get to see your partner very often as he or she lives too far away to visit on a regular basis, and most of your bonding occurs over the phone or e-mail, this doesn't mean that your sex life has to be on hold. This is when that old adage that absence makes the heart—and everything else—grow fonder holds true! You can still build sexual tension and, with your partner's help, have an amazing orgasm even though you're miles apart. Whether you're on the road and away from your partner for just a few days or you're engaged in a true long-distance relationship where months may go between the times when you're able to see your other half, you'll find the following entries useful to help you both achieve amazing orgasms together.

129. Dial Up the Excitement with Phone Sex

When you're not within touching distance, a great way to arouse your partner is by having phone sex together. After all, a certain phone company used to have a slogan about reaching out and touching another. Their intention was more innocuous, but you can certainly reach out and touch—and turn on—another with your voice. Having phone sex is similar to talking dirty, but since you can't engage in the kind of dirty talk outlined in Tip 124 unless you're in your lover's presence, make do in the meantime with some hot and heavy sessions over the phone.

A great way to get started is to ask what your partner is wearing that night and then "mmm" at the response. Even if they respond by saying something not very sexy, mmm'ing could get you both laughing and bonding. Then, when you've determined that your partner is in the mood, start your less innocent conversation. Ease into it by telling your partner how you would touch him if he were nearby, and then work up to the point where both of you are saying all of the things you would do to each other. Sighing and moaning are important in the bedroom, but they're even more important here, as your lover is only able to sense the level of your desire through what you vocalize. Eventually, you two might get so into it that each of you begins to imagine you're having sex with the other in person and describe those actions while the other person masturbates to orgasm.

130. Set the Tone by Sexting

Another popular way of turning on your mate when you're far away—or even not so far away—is by sending sexually suggestive text messages, or sexting. If you two can really get going, it can be a fun distraction while you're at the office and if you two work close enough, you might decide to meet up for a midday rendezvous!

However, if you send one such as "just thinking of you and getting wet," and you don't get anything back, don't worry that you've offended your partner. Some people just aren't big texters, or your partner might not know how to respond. If you've sent a couple flirty or sexy texts and you haven't gotten much of a response from your partner, talk to them about their opinions on sexting. It may turn out that they're not super into it, but maybe they're just shy and need a little encouragement.

Another option, if texting isn't your style or you're particularly into the written word, is to exchange sexy e-mails. The e-mails don't have to be long, but make sure to express the dirty thoughts that are running through your mind to make your partner eager to get back to the bedroom.

131. Experiment with Cybersex

Cybersex is similar to phone sex, but the interaction occurs over the computer, as it involves typing your desires to the person on the other end. This can be done over any instant form of online chat. There are also a handful of online programs that let you create an avatar and allow your avatar and your partner's to engage in a variety of sex acts together. To spark a fun session, try some of the tips I've outlined under "Dial Up the Excitement with Phone Sex" (Tip 129) and "Set the Tone by Sexting" (Tip 130). Just be mindful not to engage in cybersex at the office. That's a great way to get fired!

132. Write Erotic Letters

In this digital age, it's hard to imagine that people still write letters. But they do, and it's almost always a pleasant surprise to open the mailbox and find a letter. Especially if it's one from your partner. If do you choose to handwrite a letter (very romantic of you!), consider upping its erotic qualities and writing your own erotic story about the two of you and what you might want to try out when you do see each other. Ask them to write you one in return so that you can enjoy pleasuring yourself to it in their absence.

133. Try Video Chat

Those who are in long-distance relationships these days don't have it easy, but at least there are many different tools to use to not only connect emotionally with your partner but also to connect with them on a more explicit sexual level. I've spoken about e-mails, letters, sexting, and phone sex, but the technology that most allows us to connect with one another as if we were actually in the room together is video chat. For a relatively low fee, this technology allows you to see each other and react in real time to your partner's words, facial expressions, and more. It also makes it easy for you two to take phone sex to the next level, as you can masturbate in front of each other and bring each other to new heights of pleasure. It's the next best thing to being there.

134. Cast His Penis

If your lover is moving away or traveling for an extended period of time, consider asking him to give part of himself to you—his penis! There are many kits on the market that will allow him to cast his penis safely and then create a dildo from it. This is a great toy for you to use when you are engaging in one of the long-distance sex methods previously covered. Not only will it give you pleasure while he's away, as it's the male member you've come to quite enjoy and you know just how you can use it to help you achieve an incredible orgasm, but it will also make him feel special because you're asking for his penis to keep you satisfied. Since most men are a little concerned about their abilities in the bedroom and the size of their member, talk about a boost to the ego!

135. Reach Out and Touch Your Partner with a Remote Vibrator

The next best thing to having your partner cast his penis into a dildo is to share the gift of a remote vibrator. The way this inventive device works is that you give him the controller (which will appeal to his fun, button-pushing side) and you take the vibrator end (which appeals to your, um, love of vibrators? Just go with it.). When you are engaging in long-distance sexual play and you turn on the vibrator, he can control the strength and frequency of its pulses with the remote so that even though you're not there, he can touch you all the way to orgasm. Of course, if he's game, you two could always switch roles and he could stimulate his perineum with the vibrator as he masturbates with the other hand. He may enjoy you being in the driver's seat; and while the dual sensation (and the buzzing) will probably be new to him, he may love it!

DID YOU KNOW?

The sacred space we talked about before (Tip 57) isn't doing any good if you hardly use it. Even if your schedules are very busy, make it a point to spend some time alone together doing something fun in your sacred space. Ideally, this would mean leisurely lovemaking sessions, but it could also include quickies, massages, adult games, watching romantic/erotic movies, or whatever else you two enjoy doing together.

While it's always the most fun to use your space for things of a sexual nature, you can also use it to just be together. If you have both had a rough day, or just need some time, go into your sacred space, turn down the lights (or turn them off altogether), put some music on, light a candle, and just lay in each other's arms. Cuddling can get a bad rap sometimes, but it's one of the most intimate things you can do with another person. Hold each other and stay perfectly quiet, or speak softly about what's troubling you. Offer advice and suggestions, and accept them in kind. Once you both feel done, leave the sacred space and go about your day.

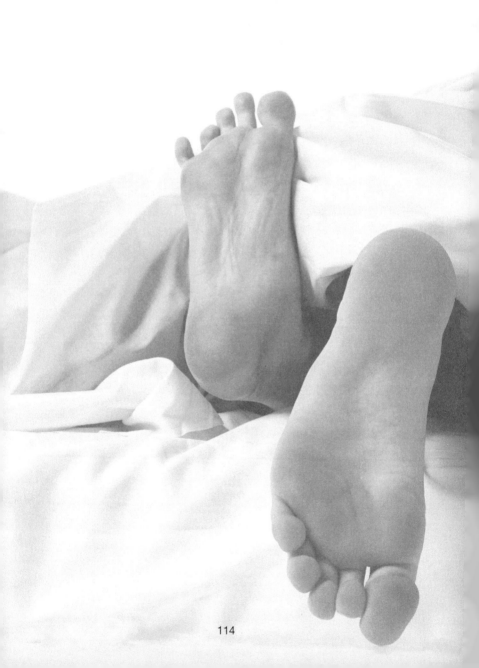

CHAPTER SEVEN

Master the Art (and It Is an Art) of Foreplay

136. Don't Skip Foreplay

For the past few tips, we've been exploring ways you and your partner can keep your sex life hot when one of you isn't nearby. But, since (or at least we hope) your partner is more likely to be around than not, let's refocus our efforts on how to really make your sex life bloom in the presence of each other. One of the most important things you can do to help improve your orgasm and your sex life in general is to not skip foreplay. While it's okay to cut right to the chase once in a while and enjoy that quickie while dinner is in the oven, cutting foreplay out most of time isn't a good idea. That's because foreplay, which involves kissing, fondling, and oral sex, is not only fun, it also brings you and your partner closer together because it allows you to really explore each other's bodies with less of a focus on getting to the orgasm. And that's a good thing when it comes to reaching climax, because the sexual tension that builds during foreplay can lead to a more intense release when that part of the night arrives. Interested in how to improve your foreplay skills? Read on for tips!

137. Kiss!

Kissing is one of the most integral parts of foreplay—and of sex. It can be a very intimate way to connect with your partner, and there are all sorts of different styles of kissing—from the quick peck on the lips to the deep, passionate kiss that takes your breath away. The latter kiss is commonly known as the French kiss (or, as the French would say, *baiser avec la langue*).

It's the type of kiss that is the most satisfying, but it's also the type that most struggle with getting right. I bet you've come across some pretty terrible kissers. But if you might be one of those who needs a few pointers, here are some tips. Pay attention to how open your mouth is and how much of your tongue you're trying to put into your partner's mouth. Ideally, it's best not to come at your partner like a frog chasing a fly or like a dog gently licking its paw. In other words, don't try to shove your tongue down your partner's throat, don't try to move your tongue as fast as possible, and don't barely open your mouth so he can't get his tongue in. You may think you're being ladylike by doing the latter, but it's just plain annoying and a definite mood killer. And please, keep the excess saliva to a minimum.

If you and your partner are compatible kissers, you're likely to get pretty turned on the more you kiss. This could eventually lead to more fun things like nibbling, biting, and everything else in the sexual canon.

But it doesn't just stop at the mouth. Make sure to explore your partner's body with your kisses—from the backs of his knees to his stomach to the side of his neck—and as you electrify his erogenous zones, you'll be sure to elicit a positive response.

FUN FACT

In the most passionate kisses, the male passes sex drive-enhancing testosterone to the female, which causes things to get more hot and heavy, which leads to more kissing, which . . . I think you know where this is going. Evolution for the win!

138. Use Your Breath

Breath can be a powerful turn-on. When your lover feels your hot breath on their neck, inner thighs, or other erogenous zones, this can heighten their sexual desire. Similarly, you can use your cold breath on places you've just kissed or licked on their body to produce an exhilarating zing. Vary it up to discover what turns your lover on the most. A well-placed puff of air can lead to a pretty breathtaking orgasm, or at the very least, put some wind in your sails to get you there!

It sounds kind of crazy, but the tingling feel of hot breath on your body can make you orgasm quicker than actual flesh on flesh, because it's the *anticipation* of touch that's getting you going. In the movie *40 Days and 40 Nights*, Josh Hartnett's character gets a girl off simply by blowing a flower petal around her body, and without touching her once, he gives her an orgasm that "blows" her away. So brush those teeth and chew some gum tonight before bed, because your breath just might be the very thing to get the next orgasm going.

139. Lick

Though the idea of licking another human being might sound strange, I'm sure you know just how pleasurable it is. After all, most sexual acts probably sound pretty odd if you just consider their mechanics. For instance, if you said to someone, "I want you to put the thing you eat with on the thing I eat with, and then I want us to move our tongues around," the likely response you'd get would be, "Um . . . why?" But that's kissing! Tangent aside, licking your partner can be a very seductive act. I'm not suggesting you bathe him with your tongue (though he may very well enjoy that), but instead, as you are kissing his body with deep, open-mouth kisses, use your tongue to tease him a bit and give him goose bumps. To do so, try tracing a line on his body, say from the navel down to the pubic bone, with just the tip of your tongue to excite him. Then blow on that same space with your hot breath.

By doing this on various parts of his body—another idea to try is running your tongue from his wrist up to his armpit to see what sort of reaction that elicits—you'll find what areas give him the most pleasure. Return to those. Again and again and again, until he's so worked up that he can't help but beg you to take things to the next level.

140. Nibble

While most people prefer not to be bitten hard, your partner may love for you to playfully use your teeth in the bedroom. As you're kissing or licking an area and you find that they seem to particularly enjoy it, try biting them gently. The response might just be "mmm." Another way to incorporate biting is through kissing. As you're engaged in a deep, intense kiss, pull away slightly. Run your tongue along his bottom lip and nibble it a little bit. More than likely, he'll moan and pull you back in even stronger. For some people, the sensation of being bitten can even cause them to orgasm or get extremely close.

If he seems to be the type who enjoys you using your teeth, try a few of the rougher techniques I mentioned in "Brush Against the Neck" (Tip 22). Just always make sure to go slow with the pressure of your bite, as it's easy to go from sexy to scary. If you're going to turn up the heat with the biting, make sure to never break the skin, as the human mouth is full of bacteria that can lead to a nasty infection.

QUICK TIP
While gently nibbling on your partner won't lead to any marks that last more than a few moments, you can accidentally give someone a hickey through biting play. So make sure your partner has a way to hide the telltale sign of passion if you're going to get super into it.

141. Scratch

Some of us think of scratching as just a way to satisfy an itch. But you can also bring scratching into foreplay as a great way to turn your partner on. Giving your partner a light, teasing scratch, or even a hard, deep one, can send good shivers throughout his body. And, while the back is ripe for scratching, other places on the body just beg for it. Start with the erogenous zones and then work your way across the body using varying degrees of pressure to see how your lover responds. Here's one technique that might send tingles up your lover's spine: Start at the wrist and scratch all the way up to the shoulder or the top of the neck. Then run your fingers through your partner's hair—most men absolutely love it when you play with their scalp—and then kiss him all the way back down.

Another great time to scratch your partner is if you're having sex or making out in the missionary position and you're on the bottom. Run your nails up and down their back—starting light and increasing the pressure if they seem to enjoy it—to ramp up the passion of the moment.

142. Pinch and Grab to Turn Your Partner On

Though you would totally get smacked in a bar for doing this to a stranger, pinching or aggressively grabbing your partner can boost desire and build sexual tension. To convey that "I've got to have you" feeling to your partner, use your fingers or your whole hand to grab onto and squeeze a fleshy part of your lover's body, such as the area of the waist right above the hip or his butt. For added emphasis, lean over and whisper in his ear that you want him . . . or if you're feeling particularly emboldened, tell him what you want to do to him when you get back home. Granted, at that rate, "back home" might be the nearest coat closet or back of the car.

Once you're in private, great areas for either of you to pinch gently include the butt, the nipples, the clitoris, and the labia, while the arms, hips, butt, breasts, and an erect penis are prime grabbing ground. Experiment to find out if you prefer being the pincher or the pinchee.

143. Touch with Fingers Only

While you're busy kissing, licking, grabbing, and nibbling on your partner, here's another technique to add to your repertoire: running your hands over your partner's entire body. During foreplay or sex, part of the enjoyable sensation stems from having their skin pressed up against yours. But taking the intensity down for a moment and just allowing each other the space to caress each other's body can heighten the level of sensuality in the act and lead to greater anticipation of what is coming next and the desire for orgasm. Also, the feeling of having someone run their fingers all across your body—or the fun of doing this for another—can be quite incredible because you never know where the caress is going to stop and what your partner is going to do next, thus helping you to reach a heightened state of arousal. One quick tip: If your partner has rough hands, ask them to use a little massage oil. Plus, that will help you two glide over each other more fluidly when you've finally reached the moment when the sexual tension can't get any stronger.

144. Play with Your Partner's Feet

Earlier in the book, I made mention of how having your feet played with can feel good and that sometimes having them touched can go beyond the point of being just relaxing to being a turn-on (Tip 34).

One way to begin arousing your partner by playing with his feet is by massaging them. This will help him acclimate to your touch in this sensitive area, especially if his feet are ticklish. Once he's relaxed, ease up on the pressure and start using gentle strokes beginning just above the calf and working your way down to the toes. Scratch the top of his feet and grab them with a lusty, desiring touch. He may be so turned on by this point that he beckons you up somewhere just a bit higher on his body.

If not, if you're up for it, try kissing his feet. You can start anywhere, but the Achilles tendon located on the back of the heel isn't a bad place to begin. Kiss the top of the feet until you reach the toes. If you want to take this a step further by sucking on the toes, it's generally a good idea to first ask your partner if that's okay, as this may be a total turn-on or a complete turn-off. But for those who like it, this can be as arousing as having their fingers sucked, as it's easy for him to mentally correlate having his digits sucked on with you sucking on another lengthy part of his anatomy.

145. Be a Tease

Just as teasing yourself as you're masturbating can create sexual tension and heighten your eventual orgasm, teasing your partner can have the same effect. Good teasing involves knowing how close you can bring your partner to a new level of excitement without pushing him over the edge. Teasing often involves touching or kissing the body and then withdrawing from the touch, and it can be particularly effective when used on the genitals. This can be done by touching the skin around the genitals and then, oops, accidentally touching them and then backing off again. Or you can try stimulating your partner's genitals by touching them at irregular intervals. Bring your partner up to the point of excitement and then back off a few times and you'll soon have your partner panting for more.

146. Undress Your Partner

We're all used to taking our clothes off. Unless you're lucky enough to get laid every night, removing your clothes can be an unexciting activity that happens just before we get into the shower or into bed. But when someone else takes off our clothes, that small act can cause big excitement. To undress your partner seductively, try undoing his pants or shirt button by button, then planting kisses on the areas you've just exposed. Run your fingers through his chest hair or over his bare chest. Men have the habit of undressing themselves in the bedroom, as they just want to get to it, so if he starts to, gently stop him and begin undressing him instead. His impatience is likely to wane and be replaced with a desire to see what move you have planned next. In fact, I wouldn't be surprised that if he didn't start with an erection when you began undressing him, he had one by the time you were finished.

147. Keep Your Underwear On

Though it's fun to be naked, it's also fun to tease your partner and yourself, and one way to do that is by keeping your panties on. It can feel a bit naughty as your partner fumbles around inside your panties, searching for those spots that will make you shudder with delight, and that will help you experience quick bursts of desire as your partner's hands trace over the part you really want touched. Plus, keeping your underwear on sends a signal that maybe you want foreplay to last a bit longer and you crave more touching of your entire body. That is, until your partner can't take it anymore and has to feel what's wrapped up down below.

But you can even try keeping your panties on during sex, as that can give the romp that "doing it before we get caught" kind of vibe that can add to the intensity.

148. Get Less Than Naked

You're attracted to your partner, but face it, you need a little variety. And I don't necessarily mean a new partner. At first, when you start sleeping with someone, seeing your partner naked is a definite turn-on. But after time, that feeling wears off, and the mere sight of them nude before you may no longer completely arouse you. To inject a little extra excitement into your sex life, keep these easy-to-find items near the place you usually make love (in case of boredom): sexy lingerie, scarves for tying up or blindfolding, and gloves. Donning these accessories—or having him do so—adds to the mood in the room, as you both know that they're intended to incite pleasure in the other . . . and lead to all sorts of new experimentation in the bedroom.

149. Make Noise

When I was giving you tips on how to achieve an incredible orgasm while masturbating, I hope I made clear how important it was to fully give yourself to the experience and not hold back. Part of that involves making noise as you pleasure yourself and when you come. So, when you're with your partner, don't get shy. Your moans will not only turn your partner on, but they're also the perfect indicators of when your partner is doing something you like and to keep doing it. Though you can also say, "Wow, that feels amazing!" (which is a nice ego boost), a simple "mmm" will probably do the trick. Also, if you're moaning and moaning but then you suddenly stop, your partner might get the hint it's time to try something new without you having to verbally express it.

That said, if you're feeling like you're focusing more on making noise than just enjoying your orgasm or the buildup to it, it's okay not to make noise just for the sake of your partner. If you know he really loves hearing you, just explain that when you get quiet, that's when you've lost your ability to speak because you're so caught up in how good what he's doing feels. I'm pretty sure he'll understand.

150. Offer a Massage

For centuries, massage has been used as a preventive medicine and a way to soothe away the aches and pains of everyday life. The power of touch is crucial to human happiness, and massage is an effective way to alleviate stress, improve circulation, and even aid digestion. If your partner has had a long day or is craving a different kind of touch than the kind that often happens in the bedroom, offer a massage. Though it doesn't seem like it would be much of a turn-on, using your hands to knead away those sore spots offers you a great opportunity to touch your partner all over, and your partner is sure to appreciate the attention. Plus, the sensual act of giving them a massage may relax them into being more ready for some action. After all, what man doesn't want their sexy partner giving them a rubdown after a rough day?

151. Amp It Up for an Erotic Massage

The same techniques mentioned here can be used during any massage, but in erotic massage there is special attention paid to turning on your lover, not just relaxing him. To prepare, light a few candles and put on some soothing or sensual music. Instrumental music or world music in an unfamiliar language is ideal, as it is less distracting than music with lyrics you could sing along with. If you have massage oil, warm it by placing the bottle in a sink full of hot water. Just keep in mind that some oils may stain, so if you're concerned about your sheets, put a towel down for your lover to lie upon. Then, follow these steps:

1. Have your partner lie face down on a flat, comfortable surface, preferably in a warm room, as it's easier for the muscles to relax when you aren't cold.

2. If you are going to use oil, pour about a teaspoon of it at a time into your hand and rub your hands together so the massage oil coats both palms.

3. Ask your partner which areas are sore or tight and request that your partner tells you during the massage if they'd like you to use more or less pressure on certain spots of their body.

4. Start with light, relaxing caresses, and as you work over your partner's body, alternate between using your whole hand and just your fingertips. Bring both hands gently down on either side of the spine and with soft, broad strokes, glide from the top of the back down to the small of the back. Then glide your hands over the small of the back, over the hips. For the return stroke, pull your palms up the sides of the body, gliding underneath the armpits (being careful not to tickle) and across the shoulder blades to the base of the neck.

5. Gradually begin to extend the strokes to cover the butt, the sides of the hips, and the arms, then move down to the legs. Starting at the ankle, glide over the calf, across the back of the knee, up the hamstrings, and over the butt. Then continue all the way up the side of the back, over the shoulder, and down the arm on the same side. Repeat for the other side, eventually covering every inch of your lover's body and adding oil to your hands as necessary.

6. Once you feel you have fully covered the back of the body, ask your partner to turn over so you can attend to the front. Begin with light caresses all over, and then put more oil

onto your hands and place your hands at one of the ankles. Start the movement by gliding over the shin and across the top of the thigh and down the other side of the leg, all the way back to the ankle.

7. During this sensual massage, allow your fingers to come close to your lover's genitals and even linger nearby, but don't actually touch them. Build up some sexual tension between the two of you by gently caressing his inner thighs, where he's going to be extremely sensitive and want you to go just a little further.

8. When his legs are fully relaxed, move on to the torso using gentle strokes around the tummy and up the sides.

By the time you're done, he'll be quite turned on and very relaxed and in the mood to make slow, sensual, passionate love . . . the type that's likely to end with an intimate, synchronous orgasm.

152. Explore Mutual Massage

Mutual massage is a very unique type of massage. It involves covering you and your lover's bodies with oil and then using your whole body—not just your hands—to move against your lover's with slow, sensual movements. It's a full-body massage given with your whole body. For this, any vegetable oil will do, but olive oil and coconut oil feel great on the skin and are excellent moisturizers. Just be sure that whatever oil you choose to use is compatible with the birth control method you've chosen. During this experience, have fun exploring each other in this new way, letting every part of your body receive attention, not just your erogenous zones. By interacting with each other in this sensual way, you'll find it could lead to a powerful, connecting orgasm.

153. Make Time for Making Love

Quickies are fun, but with all the multitasking you do in the rest of your life, it's important to make time not just for having sex but also for making love. When you carve out the time (not just in your calendar but mentally as well), it's a way to let your partner know that being intimate with them is very important to you. It also allows you both to try out new techniques and ideas for lovemaking that more rushed sex doesn't allow for. This could easily result not just in a deeper closeness between the two of you, but also new ways to bring each other more intense orgasms than either of you ever thought possible.

154. Make the First Move

Within most relationships, the guy is usually the sexual initiator. It's pretty much hard-wired into their testosterone and the instincts they've developed during their evolution. But that doesn't mean they don't love it when the woman makes the first move in the bedroom. Taking the sexual initiative is a great way to show your partner that you're interested in them sexually as well and not just having sex with them because they want to do the deed. And there's nothing that can rev up someone's desire like the feeling that their partner wants to pleasure them in all sorts of ways. Additionally, making the first move takes the pressure off of him to try and judge when you might be in the mood. So, especially if you're the type of woman who often says no, reaching over and starting something with your guy will get him excited in no time.

155. Indulge in Simultaneous Masturbation

Have you ever walked in on your partner masturbating? Was it a turn-on for you? If so, why not try it in the bedroom? There's something very erotic about watching someone pleasure themselves, and it's also a great learning experience. Watching your partner bring himself to—or close to—orgasm is a good way to learn what ways he likes to be touched. As he touches himself, feel free to join in and have him guide you so you can get the feel for the type of pressure and speed he enjoys. Or, if you've already gone through basic training, you can kiss and fondle your partner with your other hand at the same time. To heighten the experience, look into each other's eyes or at each other's genitals while you're touching yourself to build some serious sexual tension.

156. Have the Breast Sex Ever

Have you ever had a guy have sex with your breasts? For some women, this can be an incredibly arousing sensation, and it's a great way to bring your guy to orgasm if you're not in the mood for having intercourse. If, like many women, your breasts are particularly sensitive during or just before your period, this might be a good time to try it, as the added sensitivity could have the effect of bringing you to orgasm or very near to it.

The best position for this is for him to sit above your torso on his knees and lean forward so that his penis is positioned just below your breasts. If you have massage oil or some other type of lubrication, pour a little onto your breasts to decrease the friction, and then hold your breasts together so he can thrust back and forth between them. If this is new for the two of you, he may climax quickly, so make sure to direct him onto you, the sheets, or (as he may love) into your mouth.

157. Tap Into Your Primal Side

Face it, we're all animals. And sometimes, making love is just not going to satisfy us. When you're feeling particularly horny and you sense your partner is in the mood, tap into those animal emotions and engage your passionate side. Kiss your lover deeply. Push your lover up against the wall and caress him. Tear off each other's clothes. As the desire between the two of you builds, use noises like growling and moaning to express your desire as you scratch lightly and bite your lover's skin. Allowing yourselves to get carried away in the moment and doing it wherever is convenient at that moment—bed, counter, top of the kitchen table—will lead to some great memories and some hot orgasms.

158. Get Artistic with Body Paint

You might not consider yourself an artist, but you don't have to know how to draw to have fun with body paint. Pick up a body painting kit at your local sex shop or purchase one online and let your imagination go wild. Use whatever colors you think complement your partner's skin tone and have fun turning each other into visual masterpieces. Don't worry about being realistic—working in the abstract is okay! Take special care when painting the genitals so you not only impress your partner with your artistic efforts, but also arouse him to the point where he desires to see what beautiful art can be made by pressing his body against yours. You may also find that getting in touch with your creative side in the bedroom will help make each of you a little more adventurous when it comes to trying out new sexual moves.

159. Role-Play

If you want to try spicing up your love life with some new characters but you don't want to bring an actual third person into the mix, role-playing is a good way to add some variety to your sex life and bring some of your fantasies closer to reality. If you've always dreamed of doing your boss or your favorite musician or being the boss, musician, or possibly even the lead cheerleader, ask your partner to step into a role that would turn you on. After the two of you play out a fantasy of yours, you can switch positions and try out one of his role-playing fantasies, too. By pretending to be other people, it can help you both get the zing you could get by hooking up with someone new, but without the emotional complications.

160. Wardrobe Change

Once you've come up with a role that you want to play—and possibly one that you want your partner to play as well—have fun getting the costumes for it. It's like shopping for Halloween, but with a much sexier purpose in mind than the local parade or Halloween ball. Some higher-end sex shops and lingerie stores sell role-play–friendly costumes year-round, or you can make sure to pick up the sexier version of some classic fantasy roles (i.e., cop, teacher, fairy tale icon, etc.) near Halloween. And don't forget the wig! The costume is critical to looking the part, but the wig is an added touch that will make it easier for you to slip into the role since you won't quite resemble yourself when you look in the mirror. Now go remind him how he's been a bad boy.

161. Shake Things Up by Switching Roles

Most of us were born one sex or another—male or female. But just because you were born female, that doesn't necessarily mean you identify with acting traditionally/stereotypically feminine. Perhaps you lean more to the masculine gender and prefer jeans and boots to skirts and heels, enjoy being in control, and are not afraid to take the initiative in the bedroom. If you were born male, perhaps you skew more feminine and prefer to indulge yourself in activities such as reading and you often find yourself attracted to strong women who take control. If you've never considered which gender you identify most with, it can be a great identity-building exercise for both you and your partner. Then, when it comes to sexual play, try on the costume of the other side of the equation for a change. If you're used to leading and being in control, allow yourself to be vulnerable and surrender yourself to your partner. If you're used to going with the flow, step up and take charge. By switching positions—figuratively and perhaps literally as well—you'll spice up your sex life a bit . . . something that never hurts when you're finding new ways to get each other excited.

162. Indulge in Fetishes

There are literally hundreds of sexual fetishes out there—items, smells, sights, sounds, or situations that inexplicably turn someone on. It could be bare feet, the warm summer sun, the smell of leather, being dressed like a schoolgirl, or whatever. For some, their fetish is so strong that they cannot reach orgasm without being around it. But for others, these objects and experiences just make it easier for them to be aroused and for them to be in the mood to reach orgasm.

Many of these fetishes come from positive experiences that occurred during childhood that, in many instances, are too far back to remember. But, to begin to weave them into your sexual canon, break the ice by expressing your fetishes to your partner. Ask him if he'd be game for trying out a few. You might find out about a few of his and have a lot of fun together playing with this new knowledge.

163. Take Erotic Photographs

The age of Polaroids and having to develop pictures has long passed, and we're now in the era where digital cameras and camera phones rule. This makes taking nude photos of your partner even easier, as now you don't have to be the couple that dropped off those pictures at your local camera store, and you don't have to worry that some stranger has made copies of your nude photos. Of course, because they're digital, this makes it easy for them to be uploaded and shared with the world via the Internet, but you wouldn't do that, would you?

If you have a trusting partner whom you believe will keep the pics private no matter what, find a day where you two feel like being creative and take turns photographing each other nude. You can use props or just pose alone. As you both get turned on and start touching each other, don't put the camera down. Use it to take photos of you touching your partner, licking your partner, and during the actual act of sex. Save them to a hidden place on your computer and have fun looking at them later—when you're in the mood for self-pleasure or with your partner—as your own personal pornography stash. They may even jump-start another hot roll in the sheets!

164. Make a Sex Tape

If you've got a handheld camera or a device that is able to record video (most phones and cameras do), use it to videotape your partner or set it up to film both of you during sexual acts. Unless you want to capture both of your bodies fully in the nude as they do in most adult films, there's no need to have an elaborate setup that involves a tripod, though that can be helpful, as it leaves both of your hands free for exploring. For starters, just keep it simple. Tape your partner going down on you as you hold the camera. Just a word of warning: Don't accidentally leave this lying around when you're done where someone (your kids, your friends, your boss, the media) can find it. Unless you want to end up in a long, awkward conversation, or have your tape used for amusement by your friends like in *Trainspotting*, these amateur films are usually best kept in a discreet location.

165. Try Everything but the Kitchen Sink

Plenty of household objects can be used for sexual play, and one of the most popular is food. If you've never tried it, two go-to standards are whipped cream and chocolate. Have your partner lie down (trying to apply whipped cream or chocolate while standing doesn't often work very well) and then cover part of him with the sugary food. Perhaps cover his nipples with whipped cream or draw a long line down his body with chocolate? Then, using your tongue and your lips, seductively eat it off of him.

And, if it sounds like fun to you, you can have him try inserting some foods into your vagina—particularly rigid items like cucumbers and long carrots. Just slap a condom on those veggies first, as you don't know how many people have handled them. Another way to use food is by blindfolding your partner and having him guess what food you're going to feed him by smelling it and feeling it. This will help heighten your partner's senses and make him curious for what you're going to treat him to next. Perhaps you can treat him to a bite or lick or some part of your body you want him to taste?

Just a few words of caution: Don't insert objects that might get lost in cavities and send the two of you on a trip to the emergency room. Also, avoid using anything sugary near the vagina, as it can lead to nasty yeast infections.

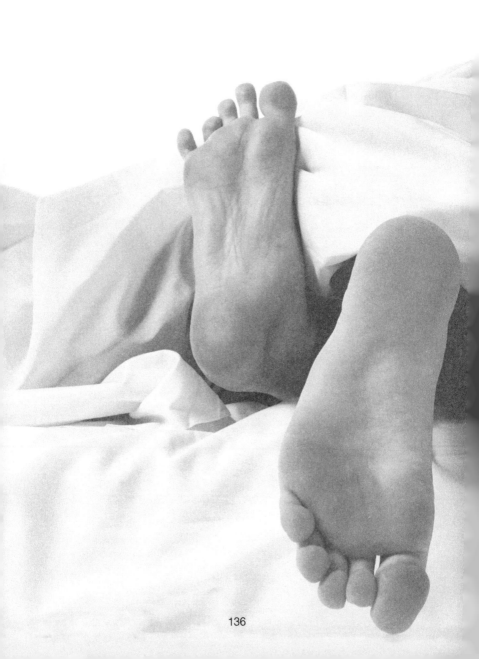

CHAPTER EIGHT

Get Yours, Girl!

166. Have Him Bring You to Orgasm Without Penetration

Getting a woman to orgasm doesn't have to be difficult. Though there are whole books written on the subject, making the female orgasm seem as difficult to crack as the Rosetta stone, it isn't. You know this. I know this. But for a lot of men, the female orgasm seems like it might as well be a myth.

There is a misconception that orgasms need to come from the act of vaginal sex, and this is just not the case. That said, for most women, getting us to reach orgasm does require a few basics: a connection between you and your partner, a reasonable modicum of attention to the clitoris, good pacing, and a partner who is capable of paying attention to how sensitive you are and which parts of your body are the most sensitive. Honestly, it's not really all that different from what a guy needs to come. They've just become very efficient at pleasuring their external organ, and the female vagina seems more mysterious since much of it is hidden. You know what you like. Share it with your partner.

Since each woman has different needs and methods by which she prefers things to happen, it's important to take the time to show your partner what works for you. Do you find it easier to reach orgasm when he's fondling your breasts? Do you prefer he leave your clitoris alone and stimulate other parts of your vulva? Your body is its own unique machine. Have fun showing him the ropes that you know can lead to the best orgasms and he'll be more than happy to follow.

167. Use Lubrication

When it comes to getting turned on, you've probably noticed that it's hard to go from zero interest to fully aroused in a matter of moments. Men, on the other hand—it takes them what, seconds? Even though we might want to go from *ho-hum* to *oh yeah* immediately, our bodies take a moment or two to catch up. This means, if you're into the idea of having spontaneous quickies, make sure to always have a little bottle of lubrication on hand to decrease the friction between you and your man when the moment strikes. Also, I should probably give you the heads-up that as you age, your body produces less lubrication—and can produce significantly less postmenopause. So if you're nearing that stage in your life, it's a good time to start to try out some different lubrication methods and find which ones feel best for you.

168. Have Him Explore the Clitoris

The clitoris has already featured prominently in this book; but as you're going to entrust its handling to your partner for the moment, I recommend you hand the book over to him for the next few tips so he can learn a few things before he begins.

Hey there, partner. So, as you're clearly keen on turning your girl on and helping her to have an amazing orgasm, I want to provide you with a few pointers. First off, do try pressing the clitoris and trying to rev her up before you've gotten her turned on. Your gal is most likely to squirm away from you, especially if your hands are dry or she is. However, after you've gotten her aroused with a little foreplay (might I suggest kissing and nibbling on her neck, ears, and caressing her shoulder blades?), start by stroking her clitoris's hood with slow, gentle strokes, using lubrication— saliva or water-based lubricant—if necessary. If she seems to enjoy this, press a little harder and start to try different amounts of pressure, teasing it by backing off and then increasing the pressure again and also by removing your hand altogether. Do it right and you'll have her moving into your hand, eager for more of your touch. Keep going and you can bring her to an intense climax without even penetrating her.

169. Step Inside

So, by now, I imagine that you've gotten your partner quite turned on by stimulating her clitoris and you may notice by now that her body is providing its own lubrication. Now is the time when you can move your fingers inside her vagina. One of the best positions for this, so you can continue to put pressure on her clitoris and her pubic mound, is by lying next to her and reaching your hand down toward her vulva. This is a very intimate position, as it allows you to kiss her and also allows her to touch you while you're fondling her. Just try to not get too distracted by her attempts to turn you on that you lose sight of your goal—bringing her to orgasm with your fingers.

Start by playing with the opening of her vagina, teasing it and making her anticipate the penetration before you actually move your fingers inside. Once you think she's ready or can't take waiting anymore, reach a finger in and move it slowly in and out of her vagina, angling your finger toward her navel when it's inside her. Continue to do this, moving your finger around inside of her, taking it out every so often to stimulate her clitoris, and putting varying pressure on her pubic mound and clitoris when you're inside. As you do, listen to the sounds she makes and pay attention to the movements of her hips. Is she trying to move away from your hand when you move it in certain ways? Does she moan if you go near her G-spot? Experiment with different strokes and pressures to see what she likes. Don't be afraid to ask her to move your hand in a way that feels good to her so you can learn what she does when you're not around and what makes her come.

170. Insert Multiple Fingers

If your partner is enjoying you fingering her clitoris and vagina, the next step before penile/sex toy/strap-on penetration is to try stimulating her with more than one finger. The best time to try this is after you've already turned her on by playing with her clitoris and using one finger inside her. The vagina is an incredible organ that is capable of stretching to allow a human being to pass through it or shrinking to make even smaller penises fill all of it. That's one of the real reasons that size doesn't matter—the vagina will adjust.

When you're trying to get her to come by using more than one finger, though, it's important that she's aroused enough that the vagina expands easily and is well lubricated on its own or with a significant amount of water-based lubricant. Multiple fingers can be painful, but if she is wet enough, she might very well find that added pressure of more fingers against her vagina's opening, where most of the nerves are, can make her orgasm almost instantly.

171. Fist for Pleasure

If your woman is enjoying having multiple fingers inside of her and you both want to move to the next step—fisting—this will require *lots* of lubrication. No matter how naturally wet she gets, get the bottle of water-based lubricant. This is also a great time to remove any jewelry you wear on your fingers and put on a latex glove if you two are using that type of STI protection. Position your hand so that your knuckles are facing her back and go very slowly, inserting one finger at a time. As you insert each, take the time to bring her close to orgasm. This will help her vagina expand and allow you to insert more fingers without causing her discomfort.

Once you've added three, the easiest way to insert the fourth is to squeeze your hand together as if you are inserting it into a jar. By doing this, the intent is to make your hand as small as possible. If, after you do this, she is still enjoying the sensation, ask her if she would like you to use your whole hand.

If she does, than add more lubrication, ask her to take a few deep breaths, slide your thumb into the middle of your palm, and push forward slowly. To reach fully inside, you may need to turn your wrist a bit, but once your hand is inside, it will curl up into a ball or fist (hence the name). When you've reached this stage, you can leave it stationary and allow her to flex her vagina as she wishes, or you can move your hand around gently inside of her or slide it inside and out as if you were using just your fingers. What you'll find as you do this is that fisting can be very intense for some women. She may ask you to remove your hand, start crying, or she may come dramatically from the intense pleasure of it.

172. Find Her G-Spot

Ladies, are you back? Good.

Ah, the elusive G-spot. It's as legendary as the Loch Ness monster, and supposedly as difficult to find. Though some women have been able to find it during masturbation because of its location on the vagina wall, it is almost easier for your partner to find it, thanks to his angular advantage. To discover it, and with it, the potential to ejaculate, once you're turned on, have your partner insert one or two fingers into your vagina and make a "come hither" motion toward your navel once his fingers are one to two inches inside. Have him feel for a part of your vaginal wall that is ridged and swollen. To aid his search, he might want to try putting one hand on top of your pubic mound and pushing down a little bit. Once he's discovered the G-spot, have him tap on it. As soon as he does, you may feel like you have to pee, but fight through that urge. As that feeling dissipates, you'll likely find that you are suddenly brought to a gushing orgasm, perhaps more intense than you've ever experienced.

FUN FACT

In 2012, more evidence surfaced that the elusive G-spot actually exists. Researcher Dr. Adam Ostrzenski published a study revealing he had found the structure during a dissection and described it as a small, "bluish, grape-like" cluster that is protected by a membrane within a sac on the vaginal wall. Of course, the presence of this structure within one person alone does not prove it exists for all women, but here's hoping it does.

173. Ease Into Cunnilingus

Cunnilingus, the act of pleasuring a woman with your lips and tongue—also known as eating a woman out—is an intimate way to bring her to orgasm. It comes from the ancient Latin words for vulva (*cunnus*) and tongue (*lingua*). As a woman, you might feel shy about letting him dive into the depths below with his mouth, but don't be. As long as you've showered that day, don't worry about your taste or smell. While it may be a turn-off to you, most men find the aroma and taste of your natural juices extremely arousing. If you're skeptical, just ask him while he's doing it if he's enjoying himself, and you're likely to hear him purr back "mm-hmm . . . " Since so many women find it easier to reach orgasm by having their clitoris and other areas in the vulva (other than the vagina) stimulated, by relaxing into oral stimulation, you may have some of the best orgasms of your life.

174. Learn the Basics of Cunnilingus

It's time to hand the book to him again as, no matter how many yoga classes you do, you're never going to be able to go down on yourself. That said, if you have a female partner, keep on reading!

Getting a woman to reach orgasm through cunnilingus can be very effective if done right, but it's also more difficult than stimulating her manually because with your head between her thighs it's hard to see what her face is doing. Here's a hint: If she pushes her vulva closer to your mouth or moans, you're on the right track. As you start, lick and suck gently around the whole vaginal area, paying special attention to the clitoris and the edge of her vagina where most of the nerves are. Then, try sucking gently on her clitoris and flicking it gently with the tip of your tongue, or inserting your tongue into her vagina. It's most likely the stimulation of her clitoris that will send her over the edge, and feel free to add pressure with your tongue and lips as you work to find out what she loves. If she grabs your head or gyrates her hips toward your mouth and you can feel her trembling and close to orgasm, don't pull your mouth or tongue away until she reaches climax.

175. Try Spelling the Alphabet

Once you've found some ways to bring your partner to orgasm with your mouth and tongue, here's another movement you might want to try. Experiment with spelling out the alphabet—upper- or lowercase letters (or both!)—with the tip of your tongue either on the opening of her vagina or on her clitoris. This technique will help you discover which part of her clitoris is the most sensitive, as the way the nerve endings are gathered on the clitoris is different for every woman. Once you find a letter she seems to enjoy, continue to repeat it until you get her to come or she's moaning for you to do something more.

176. Make Figure Eights with Your Tongue

Another cunnilingus technique she might enjoy is for you to make figure eights with your tongue on the opening of her vagina or her clitoris—which one you choose really depends on which makes her eyes widen more. Like with the alphabet maneuver (Tip 175), this movement will help you determine what part of her clitoris is the most sensitive, though typically most of the nerve endings are located in the ten and two positions if you're looking at the clitoris as a clock, with six closest to her vagina and twelve closer to her navel.

177. Add a Finger (or Two) While Going Down

Some women prefer external pleasure to being penetrated, while other women can't reach orgasm without penetration. That's why there are all sorts of different types of vibrators, from those that just stimulate the clitoris and other external parts of the vulva to those that she can use to penetrate her vagina deeply. If she is the type that prefers both internal and external stimulation, the next time you're going down on her, try inserting a finger or two while you're sucking and licking her clitoris. The combination of fingers and tongue, especially if you're stimulating her G-spot, can lead to an orgasm quicker than you'd expect.

178. Try Tribadism

Typically this act, more commonly referred to as scissoring, most often describes the sexual act of one woman rubbing her vulva against another woman's. But it can also refer to your pressing your vulva against an inanimate object or another part of your lover's anatomy, such as a thigh. As I've mentioned, many women can reach orgasm through clitoral stimulation alone, and because tribadism is focused on stimulating the clitoris, it can be a very effective way of bringing you to orgasm. While many lesbian couples enjoy this act of sexual stimulation, don't be shy to give it a chance with your man either by "dry humping" before you're ready to have sex or bringing yourself to orgasm by rubbing and pressing on a meaty part of his body.

179. Don't Forget the Rest of Her Body

If he's been busy pleasuring you down below, he may become so focused that he accidentally begins to neglect the rest of your body. Don't take it personally—he's just trying to help you see stars. If you want him to pause for a moment, just gently guide him away from your vagina and lead his mouth and hands to other parts you want stimulated. If he finds that taking a break from your vulva and kissing and licking your other erogenous zones is a good way to build sexual tension and heighten your arousal, he'll learn to incorporate this into his method. However, if you're close to reaching orgasm but want your legs, arms, stomach, or breast touched to really put you over the edge, just take his hands and move them to those areas while you continue to caress the top of his head. Doing so will help him get the hint that you don't want him to stop until you've finished.

DID YOU KNOW?

Attention, ladies and their loving partners! Every woman's body is unique and different. You know your own body best, especially if you've made self-exploration and examination a regular routine. This goes for partners, too! You know your lover's body pretty well, or are on your way to knowing it well. Examine your partner's body today, running your hands along her skin. Make mental notes of what you see (and if you do anything that seems to be turning her on!); this way you'll get a good idea of what is "normal." Plus, there are certain parts of her body that your lady couldn't see even if she wanted to (without the benefit of a good mirror, anyway!), including her back, her vulva, and her anus. Plus, your partner lives in her body and sees it every day, so having an extra set of eyes (and hands!) can really help.

Among other benefits, one good thing about this is that you will be able to quickly spot anything new or unusual. Certain fluctuations and changes are normal and expected, especially as monthly cycles come and go. But anything that just doesn't look or feel right warrants your attention. This would include any rashes, sores, tender spots, or areas that suddenly become painful. Cysts or lumps also need to be taken seriously. Don't panic right away; many of these things can be totally normal and harmless, or easily treated. However, if it is something potentially serious, the sooner you consult your doctor or seek treatment, the better off you will be.

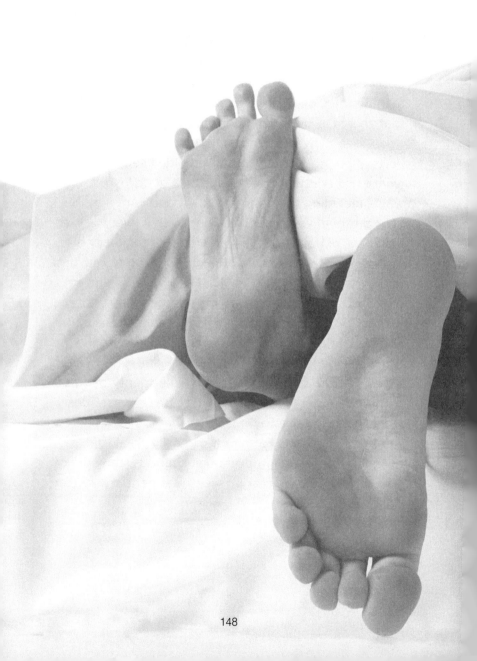

CHAPTER NINE

Get Him Off

180. Bring a Man to Orgasm Without Penetration

Now that we've spent some time exploring how a man can pleasure you and help you to have some pretty amazing orgasms, it's time to return the favor and help him have some mind-blowing ones, too. To be fair, it's pretty easy to make most men climax, but some have trouble achieving orgasm without vaginal (or anal) penetration. But, like women, while men also enjoy being pleasured manually and orally, they crave a little mental stimulation to arouse them before you take things to the next step.

What are some great ways to do this? As you've learned, men respond well to visual stimulation, so wear something sexy and flirt with him to get him turned on. Tease his body using your hands and lips to build up the sexual tension between the two of you, and run your hands and mouth over areas close to his genitals like the inner thighs to have him bending his hips toward your touch. When he finally looks as if he just can't take it anymore, begin touching the penis and testicles directly. If you're the type who can enjoy the pleasure of others, nothing will turn you on like making sure your man gets off.

181. Lube Up!

Men don't really complain about sex. They're usually pretty happy as long as they're getting it regularly. But if there's one complaint I've heard the most, it's that their partners don't use enough, or any, lubrication when they're touching their penis. Though they find the initial sensation of being touched with someone's hand extremely arousing, because the penis is not naturally self-lubricating, the friction quickly gets to be too much, and the feeling of pleasure is replaced with one of pain. To avoid this when you want to give your man a hand job, make sure to use enough lubrication so your hand can slide easily along the shaft. You can either use your own saliva or, preferably, some water or oil-based lubrication so that things stay wet the whole time.

182. Learn the Basics of a Hand Job

Manual stimulation of the penis—more commonly known as a hand job—is fairly straightforward. Men love to have you stroke it, and for most to reach orgasm, wrapping your palm and fingers and sliding up and down his shaft and over the very sensitive head of their penis using a rhythm that increases in pressure (and sometimes speed) will make them come. Just one note: A lot of men are concerned about the look and size of their penis. So if you find his penis attractive, or the skin of the shaft soft, or its size turns you on, don't be shy to tell him so.

183. Have Him Guide You

Most men know exactly how they like their penises to be touched. After all, many have been masturbating since they were teenagers, and they seem to have it down to a science. But, like you, every guy has his particular quirks and turn-ons when it comes to doing what it takes to reach orgasm, and if you're having trouble getting a grip on just what he enjoys, the easiest way to learn is by having him show you. After your hand is well lubricated, place it on his shaft and ask him to put his hand over yours and show you a rhythm and pressure he enjoys. You can ask him to do this until he orgasms (which you might find to be a turn-on yourself) or until you think you've gotten the hang of how he likes it. Either way, you'll soon find which parts of his penis are the most sensitive and pleasurable to the touch for him. But that doesn't mean you can't use a few of the following tips to get him moaning for more.

184. Switch Hands

Because of the way the vagina is constructed, it's difficult for either you or your partner to find a good angle using both hands. Usually one hand or another will feel better. But, because the penis is external, you can switch hands during a hand job to enhance the sensation.

Try making a fist with one hand and slowly sliding the head of his penis through the space as you move it down the shaft to the base. Just before you lift your hand off, place your other hand on the tip and start again. The motion you're aiming for is a continual one, almost as if you were milking his penis in reverse so it provides the sensation of penetration. Then, switch directions and see which method he prefers. By moving your hands upward, you'll tug on his foreskin—or what remains of it—which may feel extremely pleasurable to him. Usually one of these two will have him moaning in near ecstasy.

185. Try the Hot Potato Maneuver

Another hand-job method to try is gently tossing his erect penis between the palm and fingers of your hands as if it's a hot potato. The idea here is for the sensation and anticipation to build up between touches. Don't be surprised if he eventually grabs one of your hands and wraps it tightly around his penis so you can bring him to climax.

186. Add These Stimulating Ideas to Your Collection

In addition to those two methods, there are countless ways to stimulate the penis. Here are some more common—and some not so common—techniques you may want to experiment with.

- Play with just the head of his penis, lightly squeezing the coronal ridge with your fingers. Then tease him by circling around it and the frenulum with one finger and using feather-light upward strokes.
- Avoid the head of his penis for a while, teasing him until his anticipation heightens to the breaking point and he's straining for you to touch the glans.
- Use the palms of your hands and your fingers to do a light corkscrew motion spiraling down the shaft and head of his penis. You can also apply this method during fellatio if you hold your hand around the bottom part of his shaft and use your mouth to corkscrew up the top and over the head.
- Use one hand to firmly grasp the base of his penis and the other hand to stroke the shaft and head.
- Use both hands together so that his penis feels totally engulfed, as if it's inside you and not just your hands. You can use this technique with any of the techniques above except for the hot potato.

187. Vary the Pressure

As you're giving your lover a hand job, it's important to vary the pressure. While the rhythmic stroking of his penis feels incredible, what you want to do with a hand job is to mimic the feeling of him being inside you as best you can using your hands. And when you're having sex, the vagina contracts and moves around his penis. Try to replicate this feeling with your hand by squeezing and releasing as you move up and down the shaft and over the glans. As he nears orgasm, keep the pressure on, as the added friction will add to the intensity of his release.

188. Navigate the Uncircumcised Male

Though many men in the United States are circumcised, the practice of removing the foreskin isn't popular all around the world, and there is a growing trend in the United States of leaving it intact. If your lover still has his, you can use all of the previously mentioned techniques, plus one more. As you're giving him a hand job, slide the foreskin up over the head of the penis and bring it back down again. The sensation of having the foreskin brought up and over the glans and back down again may drive him wild. In men, the foreskin is analogous to the clitoral hood, and you may find that the glans of uncircumcised men is more sensitive than those of circumcised men. If that's the case, then stimulating the glans through the foreskin itself when you're touching it with your hands may be more pleasant for him.

189. Finesse Fellatio

Fellatio—like *cunnilingus*—comes from Latin. In this case, from *fellare*, meaning "to suck." Also like cunnilingus, this practice— known more commonly as a blow job—involves using your mouth and tongue to help your lover reach orgasm. Men love the act, not just because there is something inherently masculine about having you pleasure them, but also because if done well, it feels an awful lot like sex. If you're not a huge fan of giving head, then read on for some pointers on how to make the experience more pleasant for you as well as how to give him an orgasm so good that his eyes roll back in his head.

190. Learn the Basics of a Good Blow Job

For your lover, the sensation of having your warm and wet mouth gliding over his penis is intensely arousing, especially because, as I mentioned, when done right it can feel almost just like the act of penetration.

Before you begin, find a position that is comfortable for both of you (i.e., not with your elbow propped on his inner thigh). Depending on your lover's sensitivity—and your technique—you might be down there for a while. Feel free to take short breaks if your jaw starts to cramp.

When you begin, start at the tip by tracing around the head and glans with the tip of your tongue, and then use your whole tongue to work your way slowly down to the base of the shaft. Depending on how big his penis is, you may have to balance the rest by holding it with one hand. Repeat this movement a few times before putting more of his shaft into your mouth.

When you feel him getting more aroused, take the head and as much of the shaft into your mouth as you can. As you move downward, try to suck a bit on his penis by contracting your mouth, and run your tongue up and down the shaft. This may take some practice to do without using your teeth. Go down as far as you can, and then back up to the head.

Then, tease him a little bit to stave off his orgasm for a moment and make it more powerful when you finally take him there. You can do this by removing your mouth and just running your tongue over the head again, using your mouth to blow warm air over his penis, or just slowing the speed and pressure down until he's begging for you to keep going. Once he's close to orgasm, keep the rhythm steady and increase the pressure. Though many men announce that they're going to come, if he's not one of them and you would prefer not to have him ejaculate in your mouth, ask him to let you know when he's about to let go. Then remove your mouth and finish bringing him to orgasm with your hand. If you are comfortable having him come in your mouth, you can then decide whether to swallow or spit it out discreetly.

191. Turn Your Mouth Into a Vacuum

Just like every woman is unique in the way she prefers to be pleasured orally, men also have their preferences when it comes to oral sex. Most men love it, but some prefer a more gentle approach while others must feel intense amounts of pressure during the act to reach orgasm. If your lover is one of the latter, make sure to incorporate intense sucking motions into your routine and keep a strong grip on the rest of his penis if you can't fit it all into your mouth. If you're not sure how much pressure your lover prefers, try varying the pressure with your mouth and hand. Just ask him to let you know if anything you're doing for him is uncomfortable so he doesn't just grin and bear it.

192. Don't Forget the Corona!

In case you missed the memo the first time, I'm not talking about the beer. When you use your tongue to trace along the coronal ridge—the largest part of the head of the penis (and the most sensitive)—expect him to respond by moaning or grabbing as a way to nonverbally ask you to keep going. Because stimulating this area is similar to him licking your clitoris, do it long enough and you might bring him to the brink of orgasm.

193. Try Deep Throat

The term *deep throat* came into the everyday lexicon following the Watergate trial and the classic adult film of the same name starring Linda Lovelace. But the concept of deep throating has been around for much longer—probably since the dawn of mankind. It involves taking the shaft of your guy's penis entirely into your mouth, all the way down to where it reaches the pubic bone. To do this successfully, you'll have to find a way to control your gag reflex. This will probably take some practice. Get into a position where you can go down on him by either lying on your side or lying with your head just over the bed. These positions help the muscles relax, more so than if you were kneeling or hovering over your partner. Go slowly, and if you're feeling as if you're going to vomit, pull back a bit.

It may take quite a few tries to be able to deep throat comfortably, especially if your man is well-endowed, but once you've got it down, it'll blow his mind.

Until then, you can replicate the feeling of being completely enveloped in your mouth by wrapping your lubricated hand around the base of the shaft as you go down on him and moving it with the same speed and pressure as your head.

194. Don't Use Your Teeth!

Unless your partner asks or has a penchant for being bitten, do your absolute best to avoid using teeth anywhere on the penis. Because the organ is so sensitive, feeling your nails or teeth on his penis can be extremely painful and can kill the momentum toward orgasm. One of the most effective ways to avoid this unfortunate occurrence when giving a blow job is to cover your teeth with your lips—if you're going down on his shaft so far that you think it would be otherwise unavoidable. If your lover *does* want to be bitten, do so gently and playfully as if you were barely touching him, and stick to nibbling on the shaft, not the head.

195. Play with His Testicles

While you're giving your partner a hand job or blow job, why not use your other hand to play with his testicles? Though the testicles are very sensitive, most men enjoy them being fondled, tugged on gently, or sucked. Doing so may cause him to reach orgasm more quickly, so just be mindful of that if you're trying to make the act last.

Want him to have a truly memorable orgasm? While you're giving him head, lubricate one hand, wrap it around the shaft of his penis, and stroke it with the same intensity and speed. Simultaneously, take the other (dry) hand, and gently massage and tug on his testicles. That's one technique he'll be asking you to repeat again and again.

196. Push On His Perineum

Most men have experienced what it's like to have their penises fondled and their testicles slightly tugged on, but some—even when masturbating on their own—haven't ventured as far down as the perineum. While you're giving him a blow job or a hand job, reach below his testicles and gently massage that space just below them. You should be able to feel a small lump just a bit underneath the surface. This is his prostate gland, but it also doubles as the male G-spot. While you can't stimulate it directly through the muscle, massaging it in this way while you're stroking his penis with your hand or mouth can bring him waves of uncontrollable desire and release.

197. Stimulate His Prostate

For most men, stimulating his prostate/G-spot by massaging his perineum is as far as they're interested in going. But if your guy is adventurous—and you're willing—give him the orgasm of his life by stimulating it directly. To put it bluntly, this means you've both got to be ready for you to stick your finger in his butt.

The best time to try this is when he's already very turned on. So, when he's aroused, cover your finger with a condom (or, if you're really brave, go in without one), and make sure to cover it in a lot of silicone-based lubrication (it works better for anal play than water-based lubricant). Then, with your palm facing upward and with him lying face up on the bed, slowly push your finger into his butt with your finger pointing toward his navel. As you're doing this, remind him to relax, as it'll make the experience much more pleasant.

What you're looking for is a chestnut-sized organ about two inches inside of him. When you find it, alternate between stroking it with a "come hither" motion and pushing gently on it to see which technique he prefers. Just be ready for his explosive orgasm.

198. Have Him Stand

To help your partner achieve an incredibly strong orgasm, have him stand—either unsupported or leaning against a wall—as you give him head either by lying on the bed, sitting on a chair, or kneeling in front of him. As he begins to get to the point where he's close to coming, he'll start to feel his knees buckle. This combination of his mind being thoroughly distracted by the feeling he's about to come but also the need to focus on standing so he doesn't collapse will result in a powerful eruption.

199. Try 69-ing

If you're the type that likes to focus on doing one thing at a time and doing it very, very well, then 69-ing might not be your cup of tea. But the erotic nature of enjoying simultaneous oral sex with your partner can help you to get carried away by your animal nature, so it's definitely worth a try at least once. Because, while it isn't easy to both give your partner head and enjoy being pleasured, it's a lot of fun.

The easiest way to have a 69 is to have one person lie on their back or side, knees down, while the other lies on top or on the side of him or her with their head toward their partner's feet. This allows each of you to easily reach the other's genitals, even if he's a lot taller than you are. As each of you gets more into it the intensity often increases, and it's easy to become aroused by feeling how close your partner is to orgasm—as that's often when he will start going down on you even more intensely.

200. Check Out Tongue Vibrators

One way to increase the intensity of oral sex without stimulating his prostate is through the use of a tongue vibrator. This gadget wraps around your tongue and has a little motor on it that produces a light buzzing sensation. It can be used anywhere on the body, but it's especially effective at causing orgasmic pleasure when used on the vulva near the clitoris or along the head and shaft of the penis. After you turn it on, begin by stimulating your partner in a less sensitive area—perhaps their thighs, side, or chest—to give them a few moments to adjust to the sensation. Then, work your way toward the more sensitive areas to induce pure bliss.

201. Have Him Sweeten His Semen

If your partner doesn't have any STIs, swallowing his semen is no big deal. But sometimes it can just taste awful. There's not much he can do about the saltiness of it, but if the taste of your partner's come makes you want to gag, he can improve its flavor by making a few adjustments to his diet just a day or two before you go down on him. When you give him the tips below, just let him know that the better he tastes, the more head he's likely to receive.

- Avoid or eat less red meat, cauliflower, broccoli, asparagus, garlic, and onions.
- Indulge in fruit and fruit juices.
- Eat vegetables and seasonings such as parsley, wheatgrass, peppermint, celery, and cinnamon.

DID YOU KNOW?

It's a cultural stereotype that sexuality comes naturally to men. In fact, many men feel stymied by cultural and family beliefs that stigmatize male sexuality. In many cases, a young man's sexual experiences begin with quick, furtive exploration. He may learn to reach climax quickly during masturbation. Then, when it comes to sexual excitement with a potential lover, his body may react too quickly. This pattern can be very difficult to change, leading to insecurity and fear of underperforming.

The male ego is very much tied to sexuality. Issues of acceptance, performance, attractiveness, and youthfulness really do matter for men just as much as they do for women. When you add to this the stress levels of modern life, things can get tough. Lack of good communication skills between couples and the changing roles of men and women compound the problem. Many people simply don't take the time to develop the skills to be great lovers.

To make a long story short, men really aren't mindless sex machines any more than women are uptight cold fish—both genders need seduction, warmth, and acceptance from their partners. Keeping the lines of communication open with your partner can make sex more fun for both of you, so always be sure to check in.

You can't expect that you or your partner will always be ready for sex. Yet many people would rather fake interest than communicate openly about their feelings. The problem with this is that it further increases the emotional distance between partners and makes great sex even less likely in the future. When you don't feel like talking much, you can simply say, "I'm not ready for lovemaking just now, but I sure would love to snuggle or spoon with you," or "I sure would love to give or receive a massage."

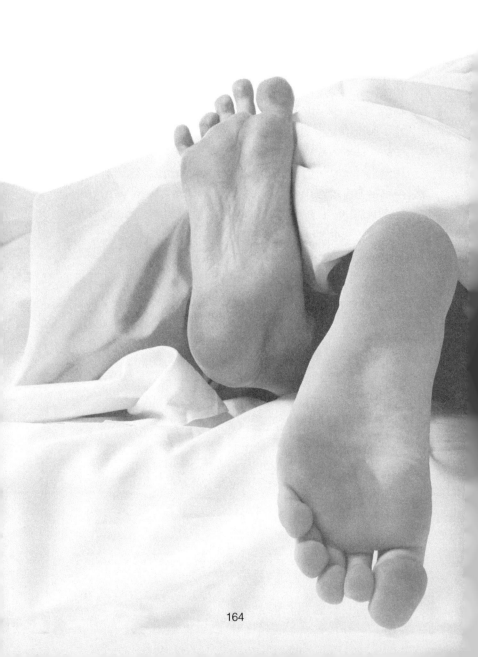

CHAPTER TEN

Achieve Perfect Penetration

202. Have Him Penetrate You

After all of this foreplay and teasing, I bet you're ready to jump into the sack (or do the horizontal mambo, make love, roll in the hay . . . whatever euphemism you prefer) and explore vaginal penetration. As you've learned from the other tips in this book, the spaces inside of your vagina where a penis can reach (but fingers and tongues cannot) are not where you're the most sensitive. But that doesn't mean that having sex doesn't feel good. The combination of clitoral stimulation—either by your partner's fingers or by his putting pressure on it through his pubic bone—with penetration can result in a truly earth-shaking orgasm.

For many of the entries that follow, though I use the word *penis*, a dildo or other penetrative object can be used in its place.

203. Decide Who's in Charge

Like dancing, sex usually requires one person to lead, or at least to do most of the leading, as it's easy to fall out of sync if both people are trying to be on top. Usually with sex, one person naturally ends up initiating more of the action, though it's fun to change roles every so often to allow your partner the pleasure of being the "bottom" or the "top" instead.

However, when it comes to controlling the speed and pressure, the woman is usually the one dictating those terms. That's because while both fast and slow sex probably feel great to your partner, you might not find all speeds as pleasurable as he does. When he's inside of you, to control the motion, move your hips or try and speed him up and slow him down by placing your hands on his butt to give him some nonverbal cues about what you enjoy. Moaning when he's doing it right doesn't hurt either.

204. Load Up on the Lubrication

I've mentioned it before, and I'll mention it again. When it comes to sex, lubrication is key to having a good time. Unless you or your partner gets off on chafing or intense friction, it's going to be awfully difficult for you both to orgasm without a satisfactory amount of lube. If you're very aroused and ready for him to be inside of you, you'll probably feel that you're very wet. But if you're not quite there yet, add a little water-based lubrication to help everything slide just a little easier. And have some fun with it. Before he's ready to penetrate you, have him put a little lubrication in his hands and have him rub it over his condom-sheathed penis and then on your vagina. Always have him add a little at a time, as too much lubrication can make it hard for you to feel him inside of you and for him to feel you, too.

205. Get Ready for Penetration

At this point, you're turned on, you've added lubrication if you needed it, and you're ready for him to be inside of you. Are you mentally ready as well? The first time you have sex with someone—whether you're a virgin or you're with a new partner—can be a life-changing experience for the both of you. The intimate act will (almost) undoubtedly alter your relationship and hopefully bring the two of you closer together. If it's the first time, do one last check to make sure you're happy with where everything is going, and then let your worries go and have fun! While it's important to have safe sex (both emotionally and physically), thinking too much about sex during the act can prevent you from having those amazing Os I've been talking about.

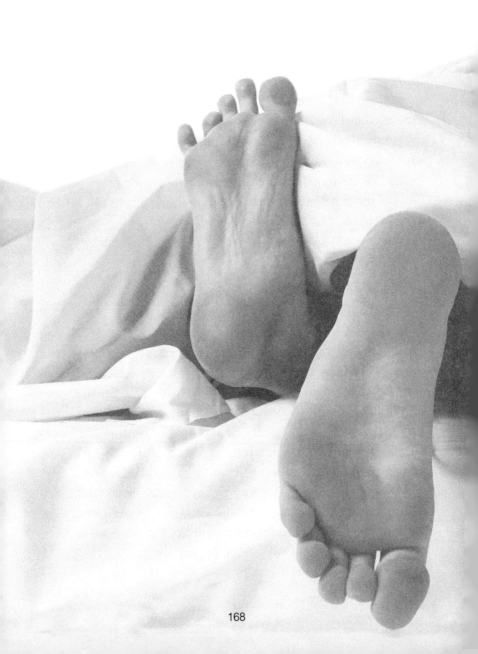

CHAPTER ELEVEN

Assume the Position(s)

206. Get Into Position

Were you one of those who, upon picking up this book, flipped right to this section? Think you're too good for all of my other handy tips? Are you already some sort of sex god or goddess who only needs a quick refresher on some of the best positions in which to reach orgasm? It's okay, I did the same thing when I first saw the *Kama Sutra*.

You'll be happy to discover that in the next few tips, I'll tackle many of the basic positions you'll want to try with your partner. Use these as jumping-off points that can add variety to improve your sex life, and alter them as you see fit. Then I'll follow these with some positions that are a little more advanced to help you and your partner find news ways to orgasm together after you've exhausted all of the basic moves. Feel free to flip back to the earlier sections if you think you need a quick reminder on a certain tip.

207. Master the Missionary Position

This is the standard, tried and true sex position you've seen in countless films, suggestive advertisements, and works of art. It is also viewed as a "boring" or "traditional" position, which could not be more wrong!

In this position, coined by sexologist Alfred Kinsey thanks to his misunderstanding of an anthropological text, you lie on your back, either with your knees bent or straight, while the man lies on top, facing you with his legs between yours.

But despite all the jokes made about how dull this position is, there's a reason Tuscans have nicknamed this *la posizione angelica*, or "The Angelic Position": It's one of the best when it comes to stimulating your clitoris and for encouraging intimacy between you and your partner. That's because the man can hold himself up with his arms in order to penetrate you deeper or, if he chooses to make the act more intimate, he can wrap his arms around you and pull you close.

Either way, the positioning of his penis and your vagina make this position a go-to for a good orgasm. Try a variation of it if you think it's too boring: sit up for maximum penetration, or rest your ankles on his shoulders rather than wrapping them around him. The impact will have you wondering why you ever questioned "The Angelic Position" in the first place—it is just heavenly.

FUN FACT

Ancient Greek diviner Artemidorus Daldianus is said to have claimed this man-on-top position was the only "proper and natural one" because it affirmed man's domination over women. Um, yeah, Artemidorus, whatever you say.

208. Tilt Your Hips

The missionary position is an excellent position to start in. It's comfortable for both you and your partner, it allows for a vaginal-centric orgasm, and it allows the two of you to easily achieve a high level of intimacy. The only trouble with it is that it doesn't allow much clitoral stimulation unless your partner knows just the right angle to position his hips. If you need a little more clitoral stimulation to reach orgasm, help him out by tilting your hips so that your butt is slightly raised up. One way to do this is to bring your legs up a bit and wrap them around his back. This will allow him to penetrate you deeper and help him put more pressure on your clitoris with each thrust.

209. Break Out the Pillows

For those positions in which you are lying on your back and you or your partner desires deeper penetration, reach for the pillows. As the lovemaking gets more intense, they're just going to get in the way behind your head, so put them to good use! Take one or two and place them under your hips or underneath the small of your back to help you raise your hips a few inches higher into the air. This allows your partner to reach your clitoris more directly as he thrusts, and because of the new angle, it allows him to penetrate you deeper. This can also help a less well-endowed partner plunge deeper inside your vagina so you can experience a great orgasm that's both clitoral and vaginal.

210. Raise Your Hips

Because the missionary position is one of the most popular sex positions, there are many ways to vary it slightly. These slight adjustments can mean the difference between *okay* and *oh yeah!*, so I recommend trying each to see which one works for you.

One more very simple alternative to the missionary position involves raising your hips into the air with your feet flat on the bed (as opposed to being around him). This exaggerated angle allows for a different sensation as well as deeper penetration and may allow your partner to reach your G-spot or A-spot, depending on what angle you're holding yourself up at.

211. Get Flexible for the Indrani

This position, derived from the *Kama Sutra*, is essentially another variation of the missionary position. This one—also known as the "deck chair"—allows for greater penetration. It's ideal for those with less-than-average penises, as it allows the man to penetrate deeply without hitting your cervix and allows even a less well-endowed man the ability to stimulate your G-spot. To accomplish this, lie on your back and raise your knees until they are at the level of your breasts. If you are flexible, place your knees into your partner's armpits. This helps spread open your vagina and allows for easier, deeper entry.

212. Stretch Your Legs Into the Yawning Position

This position has nothing to do with sleep. Instead, it's yet another tantalizing version of the missionary position that is great for those who orgasm best through deep penetration or stimulation of their G-spot. To get into position, lie on your back and place your legs up and over the shoulders of your partner. Like the Indrani, this position allows for deep penetration, so ask your partner to be gentle at first.

Another benefit of this position is that it allows you to have more control over the speed. You can also impact the angle he's penetrating you at just by adjusting the position of your hips so he can connect with your G-spot (or not, if you prefer). It's an ideal position if you've been doing Kegel exercises, as you'll be able to take advantage of your ability to squeeze your PC muscle and prevent him from coming too quickly.

One slight variation of the Yawning position is this: instead of putting your legs over his shoulders, put them on either side of your head. Obviously, this is only recommended if you're very flexible, but it allows more pressure to be put on the penis and vaginal opening, which can result in a more intense orgasm, since that's where most of the nerve endings are located.

213. Rise Up Into Position

Another Yawning-inspired position is known as the Rising position. Here, you'll want to put your legs straight up so that your feet rest on your partner's chest. He can either hold onto your hips and thrust to penetrate you deeply, or you can control the movement and move your hips so he penetrates you at the speed you desire. If that's uncomfortable, place both of your legs on one side of him near his right or left shoulder, and see how that feels.

214. Split the Bamboo

A more challenging version of the Rising position is known as Splitting Bamboo. To accomplish this one, keep one leg bent at your side or flat on the bed, and put the other leg on top of your partner's shoulder while he kneels or sits on his feet. As you make love, switch the position of your legs (left foot resting on his shoulder while the right foot is flat on the bed, then vice versa) every few moments. One side is likely to feel more pleasurable to you than the other, but the switching can create a sensation that will take you closer and closer toward orgasm. Once you've got the hang of it, begin to rotate your hips so he can stimulate your G-spot.

215. Get on Top

For the last few positions, I've had you lying on your back, so let's reverse things for a moment. By being on top, you'll have more control over how deeply you want to be penetrated, the speed at which you want to move, and how much stimulation your clitoris is receiving. Plus, in this position, it makes it easier for your partner to gaze upon your gorgeous body.

A few other great things about being on top—your partner will get to take a break from thrusting and allow you to "do the work" for a moment (which he'll likely find to be a serious turn-on), and it may help to prevent premature ejaculation in partners who get off a little too quickly.

The most common variation on this position is merely the reverse of the missionary (with you on top) but there are many other variations that I'll go over.

216. Flutter Your Butterfly

One common woman-on-top position involves having your partner lie flat with his legs together or with his knees slightly bent as you sit on top of his penis almost as if you were sitting atop a saddle. To thrust, use your hands and knees—or just the strength of your legs if you have strong quads and hamstrings—to lift yourself partway off of his shaft and lower yourself back down again. Though this requires a bit of aerobic endurance to continue, the sensation created by the anticipation of each next thrust can be very pleasurable for both you and your partner. If you end up tiring out, rest for a moment while he continues with the thrusting.

Or, if you're not terribly athletic, you can try this position with your knees on the bed and lift yourself up from that position. The sensation won't be quite as extreme, but it will still be pleasant.

217. Ride Him Reverse Cowgirl Style

One variation of the Fluttering Butterfly is the Reverse Cowgirl position. To accomplish it, turn around so you are facing your partner's feet and lower yourself onto his penis. From here, you can thrust your hips in vertical or circular motions to help him penetrate you deeply. This is an amazing position for orgasm if you don't need clitoral stimulation to get off, as you can vary the angle of penetration and where the tip of his penis connects within your vagina merely by leaning back or leaning forward, resting your hands on his legs to support yourself as needed.

218. Alternate Feet

This position doesn't have a sexy name, but it makes up for that with its ability to help him reach your G-spot. In this woman-on-top position, you'll put one foot flat on the bed and place the knee of your other leg on the bed and then lower yourself onto your partner's penis. Then, begin to rock your hips. It shouldn't be long until the head of his penis is touching your G-spot. Want to pull him closer? Wrap one hand around his butt and hold it as you move.

219. Enter from the Rear

Rear-entry positions are those in which penetration comes from behind, not those that involve anal penetration (I'll get to that a little later in this book). That said, many of the positions we've already covered—and the rear-entry ones—could be used during anal sex. But, for the moment, try these positions that, as cheesy as it may sound, engage your animal spirit with vaginal penetration. If you're looking for passionate positions, these are those. In any of these positions, the man can caress most of a woman's body, and the woman can reach behind and feel his scrotum and penis as he is entering her. But they're really about getting in deep, hard, fast, and intense . . . and they all have the ability to stimulate your G-spot.

220. Begin with Doggie Style

The missionary position is the most common lying-down position, and this is the most common rear-entry position. To try it, get on all fours (on your hands and knees) while your partner kneels or stands on the ground behind you while you're on the bed. To move together and help you hold this position as he thrusts, have him hold your waist as he moves.

For a more intimate version, the man can lean forward so his head is just above your shoulder blade and place one hand on your heart and the other on your stomach so his motions are truly entwined with yours.

221. Be a Lazy Dog

After having sex for a while in the doggie-style position, it's easy to become tired of holding yourself up, and you might be craving stimulation of another part of your vagina. If this is the case, lower your head and chest to the bed but keep your butt high in the air, tilting it as skyward as you can. As you do this, your partner should move closer so that his penis is nearly directly above your vagina. By doing so, he'll be thrusting more toward your navel with each movement. This position puts intense pressure on the penis and on the opening of the vagina and can result in an intense orgasm for both you and him.

222. Make Like an Elephant

In this position, known as the Elephant, lie on your stomach with your legs stretched out while your partner lies on your back or kneels between your legs. As he holds onto and moves your hips and butt, this position allows him to penetrate you very deeply, but also allows your clitoris to be stimulated by the surface on which you're lying.

223. Play Sexual Leapfrog

This position requires a lot of balance, but it's a fun one to try. In it, you'll need to squat as if you're about to leap forward like a frog, while your partner kneels behind you on the bed. Lower yourself onto his penis, and once you find your center together, begin thrusting in one motion together until you both orgasm or fall over.

224. Invert Your Rear Entry

Another way to have fun with rear entry is by having your partner lie down on the bed with you lying on top of him. Though penetration is a bit difficult from this angle and the two of you may need to do some maneuvering to find a way to hold your hips so he can thrust without falling out, this is one of the more intimate positions for rear entry, as it allows your partner to touch all of your body as he's inside of you.

225. Stand Up

Ever heard how working out makes sex more fun? That's not just because staying fit helps men have stronger erections or because it provides greater cardio endurance that allows you to last longer in bed; it's also because it allows you to have sex in positions that require strength. Most standing positions require the man to have some degree of upper-body strength if you want him to last for more than a handful of thrusts. In the classic standing pose, you'll face him and wrap your legs around his butt and thighs as he supports you with his arms. This position can allow him to penetrate deep inside your vagina but it can also delay his orgasm, as he also needs to focus on holding you and staying upright.

If he hasn't been doing push-ups and you want to try this position, have him hold you up so that your back is pressed up against a wall or another strong, flat surface. It still won't be the easiest position for your partner to do if he isn't buff, but he'll be more likely to get in at least a few thrusts this way.

226. Have Him Stand and Deliver from the Rear

Here's a standing position most of you should be able to do. Lean against a wall with your back facing your partner and have him enter you from behind. This passionate, primal position allows his hands the freedom to glide all over your body and massage your clitoris to help you reach orgasm. If you want to feel him deeper inside of you, just lean further over, so the move essentially becomes a standing version of doggie style.

227. Get Carried Away with the Wheelbarrow

Do you remember how, growing up, you used to do the wheelbarrow? That's when you'd pick up a friend's legs and run holding them while your friend used his or her hands to move forward. That movement is the inspiration for this move, which, as you might imagine, requires you to be able to balance yourself as he thrusts. The positioning is the same as the old-school wheelbarrow, just with a sexy twist. In this version, your partner should stand behind you and hold up your legs as you support yourself with your arms. Once you're both in position—and balanced—he can begin to thrust. If you're a lot shorter than your partner, here's a trick you can try to make this position easier: get a thick book and rest your arms on it to give yourself a little lift. By positioning your hips higher, you'll find the position may be even more stimulating.

228. Screw While Screwing

In the uniquely named Screw position, have your partner kneel or stand on the floor next to the bed while you lie on your side on top of the bed with your knees pulled toward your chest. The idea here is to find the level at which his penis is at the same level as your vagina. Doing so will allow him to penetrate you deeply, and you can tilt your hips to find the most pleasurable angle and help him reach the G-spot or A-spot.

229. Sit Down

Many sitting positions, known in the *Kama Sutra* and in Tantric sex as *yab yum* (Tibetan for "father-mother"), are ideal for intimate contact and closeness between two partners, much in the same way as lying-down positions can be. And, unlike horizontal positions, you can have sex sitting practically anywhere—in chairs, on couches, on the floor, in bed, you name it. For that reason, they're also much easier to get away with in public, especially if you're wearing a skirt. The only drawback is that the positions don't always allow for the deepest penetration, but as you know by now, that's not the only way to reach orgasm.

To try the basic sitting position, your partner should sit cross-legged while you sit on top of him and face him with your legs wrapped around him so the soles of your feet touch (or come close to touching) behind his back. If he's not able to sit cross-legged, have him put his feet on the floor while you sit on top of his lap and the pair of you rock back and forth together, varying your speed as the intensity heats up.

230. Snuggle Up Like Two Peas in a Pod

This position doesn't look like any pea pod I've ever seen, but it does convey the closeness of that saying. To do it, ask your partner to sit back with his legs folded underneath him while you sit on top of him with your back facing his chest. As you lean forward while keeping your hips pressed against his, this position allows him to both penetrate you deeply and caress your stomach and breasts as he does. If you need a little balancing help, place your hands on the wall or headboard.

231. Clasp Your Partner

Most of the positions I've mentioned so far require you to spread your legs so your partner can get his penis as far inside of your vagina as possible. But in clasping positions, you want to actually keep your legs as close together as possible, as this creates an entirely different sensation and allows for more clitoral stimulation.

The basic clasping position resembles the missionary position with you on the bottom and him on top, but instead of spreading your legs, you'll want to hold them together. It's also a great position if your partner isn't very well-endowed or if you prefer him not to go very deep, and it's ideal for stimulating the vaginal opening and, if you angle your hips just right, the G-spot as well.

232. Use the Scissors

This variation on the basic clasping position begins in a similar position as the missionary-style version, but the Scissors position allows for deeper penetration. Lie on your side next to your partner with him behind you. Keep your legs together and have him get into a position so his penis is perpendicular to your vagina. Now, entwine one of your legs with his and have him begin to move inside of you. Having sex in this position should stimulate your clitoris directly, and he'll love the pressure it puts on his penis.

233. Spoon

Unless it's one of those hot summer nights, spooning is such a great position for sleeping. Curling up with your back against your partner—or with his back against you—with his arm draped over you is a close, intimate position that is ideal for snuggling. But it's also great for sex. The position allows him to touch you all over as he wraps his body around yours, and it only requires a touch of maneuvering to get his penis into the proper position for penetration. Though it's difficult for him to thrust in an intense, passionate way in this position, it does allow for slow, intense lovemaking. And, if the heat builds to that level, I'm sure you two will move into one of the more suitable positions I've mentioned.

234. Try Out the Coital Alignment Technique

Many of the missionary-style positions I've covered so far are great for helping you attain that perfect orgasm. But here's another tip to help: When you're in the missionary position, have your partner move his body about four inches toward your head. He should then begin to move his hips to thrust in a way so he's rubbing his pubic bone against your pubic mound and clitoral hood. By doing so, he'll be able to more directly stimulate your clitoris with his penis instead of just using his penis to stimulate your vaginal walls, and you can imagine how good that will feel.

FUN FACT

In a 2009 *Redbook* magazine survey, 51 percent of the female respondents said they reach an orgasm always or almost always during sex with their partner. Also, 35 percent said they never fake orgasms. Of those who do, 60 percent said they do it to spare their partner's feelings, while about a third said they do it in order to wrap up the sexual encounter.

We'll talk more about this later, but faking an orgasm, even though you might mean well, isn't doing you or your partner any favors. If you're faking it to be kind, you're not getting off, and he's not learning how to get you off—in fact, he thinks what he is doing is working! Be honest with your partner; if you're not going to orgasm, let him know that you don't think you're getting there. Then offer different ways that you might experience orgasm (such as changing position, etc.), or simply let him know that it's not happening this time.

This is also a great opportunity for you two to explore some surefire ways to seal the deal. Is there one move, trick, or position that always finishes you off? If an orgasm from sex alone is just not happening, try using an external vibrator, warming gel, or any other toy or device, or just have him touch some of your noted hot spots or erogenous zones. A quick nibble on the ear or a stroke on your breast can often be the magic touch to finally push you over the edge!

If you're faking because you want the encounter to end, stop now. Keep the lines of communication open—if you want a sexual encounter to end, tell your partner and *end* it. If you're tired, say so. If you're getting sore, definitely say so. If you don't mind continuing but know that it won't end in an orgasm, let your partner know not to expect you to have one.

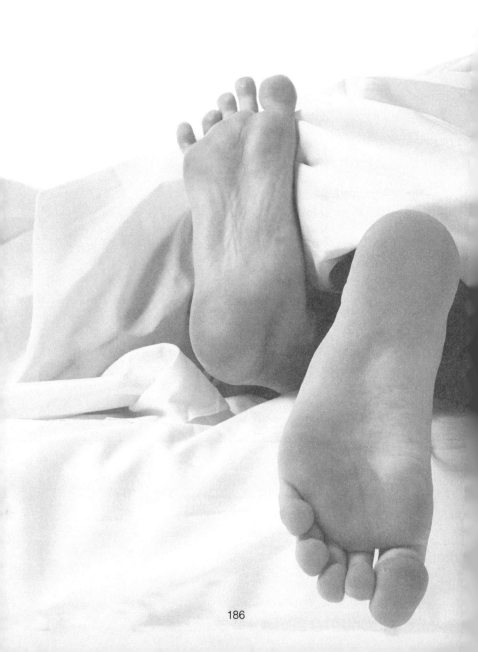

CHAPTER TWELVE

Advanced Positions for Advanced Orgasms!

235. Go for the Gold with These Advanced Positions

I've provided you with enough sitting, standing, and lying-down positions for you to have mastered the basics. You're now ready for the next level—advanced positions. The positions that follow range from just a little more adventurous or exciting to just plain difficult. Be sure you're adept at your favorite positions before trying any of these.

So, know your limits. The point of these advanced positions isn't for you to prove your sexual prowess, it's to improve your orgasms. Go slow, have fun, and don't end up in the emergency room on my account.

236. Survive—and Thrive—in the Amazon

The Amazon is a wild place, full of still-to-be-discovered flora and fauna, dangerous animals, and breathtaking plants. But you don't have to travel to the Amazon to experience a little wildness in the bedroom—just try the Amazon position. To do this, have your man lie on his back and bring his legs toward his chest so his erect penis falls between his legs. Now, straddle him and lower yourself onto his penis. From this position you can move by lifting yourself up using the strength of your thighs. Not quite strong enough for this position? Add some squats and lunges to your workout routine to build up your leg muscles.

237. Master the Twin Serpents

Even if snakes freak you out, this is a position that you might love. In it, you'll lie on your back while the man lies on top of you facing your feet so his penis is just above your vagina. After penetrating you from this position, you can wrap your legs around his back to help him stay inside. The position puts pressure on the G-spot and on his penis and that can result in an intense orgasm, but it does make thrusting difficult and sometimes can make even staying inside of you a challenge.

238. Criss-Cross to Climax

If it's been a long week and you're both tired and looking for a position that allows for deep penetration without a lot of thrusting, this is it. The Criss-Cross is essentially a diagonal version of the missionary position. To accomplish it, lie on your back and have your partner lie diagonally across your body with his legs on either your left or your right side. The pressure this position puts on the head of his penis and on the opening of your vagina is intensely pleasurable, and after a few minutes in this position, orgasm should soon follow.

239. Work the Backwards Wheelbarrow

Just in case the Wheelbarrow position I mentioned in Tip 227 wasn't difficult enough for you, try the Backwards Wheelbarrow. To do it, you've got to be a bit of an acrobat, but even if you can't hold the position for very long, it's a fun one to try. *Just please, be careful.* Have your partner face you as you wrap your legs around his thighs. Then, lean backwards so you are almost doing a

handstand away from him, using the bed or floor to support yourself as he thrusts into you.

240. Embrace Your Inner Acrobat

Did you have a childhood dream of running off and joining the
circus? Then this is the position for you. In it, your partner should
lie flat while you lie on top of him as you did with the lying-down
rear-entry position (Tip 224). Once here, tuck your feet underneath him and lie all the way back so he is deeply inside you and
your back is arched as if you're doing the Wheel position in yoga.

241. Unwind in the Armchair

If your partner has been working hard at the gym and wants to
show off his newfound strength, try this move. Ask your partner
to lie on the bed so you can get into position on top of him.
Position yourself so you're sitting on his lap facing him and place
your legs on his shoulders. Now have him sit up and keep his
back straight as he supports himself with his hands. Lean back
so you are supporting yourself with your arms as he begins to
thrust. If you're having a difficult time supporting yourself, hold
onto his waist or arms.

242. Learn How to Ejaculate

Throughout the book, I've talked about how intense a G-spot
orgasm can be. And for some women, this can result in ejaculation.
Like men, women ejaculate through the urethra and the come may

dribble out or spray. But, while it does come out of the urethra and has some of the same components as urine, it's not the same. That's because the fluid—which may result in as little as two drops or as much as two cups—originates from the Skene's glands within the vagina. Get a towel ready.

If the idea turns you on and you want to try this, first empty your bladder so that the sensation that you have to pee doesn't turn into you actually urinating. Then have your partner arouse you to the point where you're seriously turned on and your vagina and vulva are engorged to the point when you could reach orgasm. At this point, your partner should stimulate the G-spot with his fingers, tongue, or penis. While he does, do your best to relax into the sensations until your body releases with an ejaculatory orgasm. Once you've mastered this and want to take it a step further by directing the ejaculate, just work on those Kegel exercises and push on your PC muscle when you're ready to come.

243. Have Him Stimulate Your A-Spot

In the tip "Discover the G-Spot and the A-Spot Pleasure Zones" (Tip 10), I mentioned how the anterior fornix zone—also known as the A-spot—is a part of the vagina that, when stimulated, can lead to an intense orgasm. It is located just below the cervix and one of the best ways to stimulate it is by having him find a position in which he can penetrate you very deeply, preferably so he is just hitting your cervix. Once he is deep inside your vagina, have him stay there and thrust slowly so that you're experiencing continual pressure. Then, angle yourself so the head of his penis connects with the part of your vagina just below your cervix where there is a small indentation that resembles a cul-de-sac. Once you've both found it, have him continue to use slow, deep thrusts and I'm pretty sure it won't be long until you're gasping in ecstasy.

244. Have Him Stimulate Your U-Spot

The U-spot, also known as the urethral opening, is located just below your clitoris and just above the opening to your vagina. Have your partner stimulate this area by fingering it gently in a circular motion using a finger wet with his saliva or water-based lubrication. Or, if you prefer, he can use his tongue to tease the area. If you really want him to drive you wild, ask him to flick it with his tongue and go between that and licking and sucking on your clitoris. He can also stimulate it during sex if he pulls out for a moment and uses the glans of his penis to rub the U-spot before plunging back into your vagina.

FUN FACT

You might wonder why people have orgasms—not that anyone's complaining, mind you. But orgasms are, when you think about it, kind of a luxury. Humans can reproduce—and perhaps even have a fairly satisfying sex life—without having an orgasm. So what's the purpose? The most basic answer to the question of why humans have orgasms is procreation.

It's true that humans can conceive without orgasms. But it's not a matter of necessity. It's more of an incentive. To ensure that humans will continue to reproduce, nature has given us the orgasm as a sensual reward. Why would we have the drive to have sexual relations if there wasn't something very enjoyable about the act? After all, the clitoris has no biological function other than pleasure, and yet it has the highest concentration of nerve endings in the whole body.

While no two orgasms are ever really alike, nor are we able to describe each man's or woman's individual experience, we know the basic path the orgasm takes each time we are graced with the experience. The important part is that the orgasm depends on each person's capacity to feel and receive pleasure.

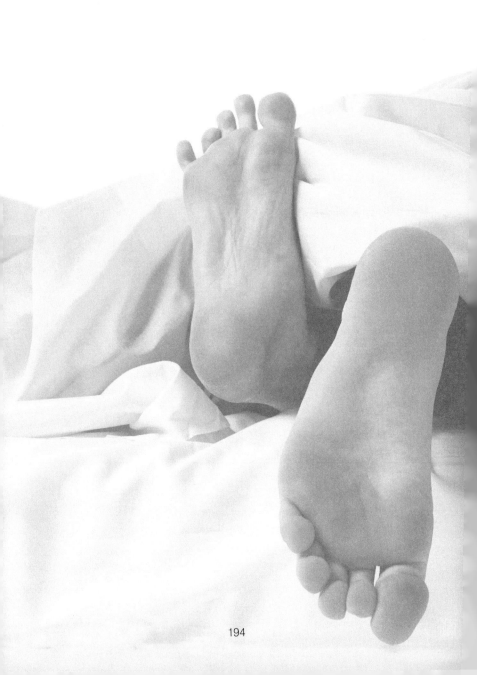

CHAPTER THIRTEEN

Be Better, Stronger, and Faster

245. Improve Your Performance

You've just learned all types of sex positions to enhance your time with your partner behind closed doors. But in addition to learning *what* positions are great for orgasms, it's important to learn some techniques that can improve even the most basic positions so that you and your partner can both experience those bite-your-lip-allow-your-eyes-to-roll-back-in-your-head moments. The next tips will help get you there.

246. Put Pressure on the Clitoris

As you've discovered through your own exploration and through the way your partner stimulates it during sex, the clitoris is a very sensitive organ. And, as your partner has probably realized, every woman prefers to have her clitoris touched differently. Some women love intense pressure directly on the clitoris, while others prefer very light, indirect pressure. Let him know how you like it—whether you want more pressure or less, prefer him to play more with the right side than the left, and so on—with verbal or nonverbal directions so he can best learn how to help you have an amazing orgasm.

247. Squeeze the Butt

You might think your partner has a cute butt, but by the time you're rolling around on the bed, I'll bet you've forgotten all about it. One way to stimulate this erogenous zone in the bedroom is, when you're close to reaching orgasm, to reach your hands around your partner and squeeze his butt to pull him closer to you. It will help him feel your orgasm—which is a total turn-on for him and a boost to his ego. One more tip: When you're close to orgasm, squeeze your butt muscles together. It'll make the feeling more intense.

248. Have Him Learn Your Body from the Inside Out

You may think you know every curve of your lover's body, but if you and your partner are free of STIs and are in a faithful, monogamous relationship where you are using hormonal contraception (or you are trying to get pregnant), have him use his fingers or his penis to explore your vagina. Have him take his time looking for the G-spot and the A-spot when both of you aren't so turned on that you're ready to pounce on one another. The knowledge gained in this fact-finding session will help you both out during other episodes, as you'll both have figured out how to position your bodies to activate your most sensitive areas. More than likely, of course, this purely recon mission will turn into anything but.

249. Watch Yourself

Mirrors are fun when we're on our own (how else could we possibly put on lipstick perfectly?), but they're even more fun when you're engaging in sexual acts in front of them. Watching your reflection as you pleasure your partner or watch him going down on you is sort of like watching porn—but with you two as the subjects—and, as a result, can be a real turn-on for both of you. And you can just imagine how exhilarating the feeling could be if you or your partner tries it while wearing a wig or some sort of other sexy disguise.

250. Dip the Tip

By now, I'm sure you know that the most sensitive part of a man's penis is the glans and the most sensitive part of a woman's vulva is her clitoris and the opening to her vagina. Here's how to really take advantage of those facts. Instead of having your partner penetrate you deeply with his entire shaft, try having sex for as long as you two can with him just inserting the tip of his penis into your vagina. When he's doing so, he can use his hand to move his penis so he can put pressure on different zones of your vagina's opening to see where is most sensitive for you (and which parts of his head and glans are most sensitive for him). This method can also be used to build up excitement, tension, and the desire to be penetrated (and for him, to penetrate) all the way.

251. Find Your Rhythm

Sex, like dancing, requires you to be in sync with your partner. And as dancing isn't going to be much fun if one person wants to rumba while the other wants to waltz, it's going to be hard to find that sweet spot where the big O happens. If you two are moving at different speeds in the bedroom. It doesn't matter whether you make love slowly and carefully, taking each moment to fully explore your lover's body and using long, slow, deep movements to construct a very intimate experience, or if you're literally tearing off each other's clothes, knocking over lamps, and doing it like wild animals. All that matters is that you're on the same page. If you're the one who is hot and bothered, try to bridle your passion until you've aroused your partner to a similar state. And if you're the one who needs a little more foreplay before sex, just reposition your partner's hands or let them know you need to be warmed up a little more if they're touching places on you that aren't quite aroused yet.

252. Be Kind to the Cervix

As you experiment with the different positions I've mentioned, you'll find that your partner is able to penetrate you much more deeply in some than in others. And while sometimes that may feel amazing, at other times of the month, it may not feel so pleasurable. During those times of the month, if he's wanting to go deep (or if he's so well endowed he can't help it), just let him know you're a little sensitive and take advantage of your vagina's ability to stretch and tilt your hips so he doesn't bang into your cervix.

By the way, in case you were worried, it's not dangerous for your cervix to be hit during sex. But depending on your body, it may or may not feel good.

253. Use Kegel Exercises to Boost Your Sex Life

Want to know an easy way to improve your orgasms? Work out your PC or pubococcygeus muscle by doing Kegel exercises. When you come, this is the muscle that oxytocin causes to contract. And strengthening it can help both men and women enjoy a more powerful orgasm.

Women, you can find it by placing the fingertips of one hand on the fleshy part of your body just above the pubic bone. Place the other hand on the bottom of your tailbone. Now squeeze as if you were trying to stop the flow of urine. The muscle you feel tensing is the PC muscle. By strengthening it, you not only enhance your orgasms, you can also tighten your vagina around your partner's penis and help yourself learn to ejaculate. Men, practicing Kegels can help you control how quickly you ejaculate and help you maintain a stronger erection (in addition to bettering your orgasm).

Commit to doing the simple exercises that follow, and you'll be impressed with how much you may improve your sex life.

254. Learn the Basic Kegel Exercises

The most basic way to activate your PC muscle is to squeeze and hold it. Like any other muscle, as you develop it, you'll be able to hold it longer and do more reps. As you do so, make sure to fully relax between each rep. One easy way to make this happen is by squeezing it with each inhale of breath and relaxing it with each exhale. Be careful not to overwork it—no matter how excited you are about improving your sex life—as you can exhaust it.

Within a few weeks of training the muscle, women may find that they can grip the penis more easily with their vaginal walls, the orgasms are more intense, and they can identify their clitoral, G-spot, and other genital muscles more easily. Men will discover that they're experiencing a greater blood flow in the pelvic region, which has resulted in a stronger erection and more of an ability to control ejaculation.

Here are four Kegel exercises to try to strengthen your PC muscle.

- Clench and release your PC muscle 20 times.
- Clench and release your PC muscle repeatedly for 10 seconds.
- Clench and hold your PC muscle for as long as you can.
- Clench your PC muscle as much as possible for 20 seconds.

255. Get a Grip on Advanced Kegel Exercises

After a few weeks of strengthening your PC muscle, you should have reached the point where you're able to do 200 reps of clenching and releasing it. Once you've reached this stage, add this to your routine: Tighten your PC muscle to the count of 10. Hold and take one long, slow breath and let it out without letting the muscle relax. When you breathe in again, tighten even harder, hold, then release your muscle and your breath after a count of 10. Work up to a set of 20. This more advanced exercise may just take your orgasms to the next level.

256. Exercise with Special Kegel Toys

It's easy enough to practice Kegel exercises without any special tools, but there are toys on the market that can help you focus on the PC muscle. The most common toys to help with Kegel practice are the ben-wa or duo-tone balls. Their weighted bearings make them particularly arousing when inserted into the vagina, and they can really help you focus on what muscle you're supposed to be working during those exercises. While you've got them in, you can do one exercise that is hard to do without—walk around with them in your vagina and work to hold them in. Doing so will definitely take some effort if you're new to Kegel exercises, but it's a great exercise to practice to tone this muscle and, with the balls inserted, one that may bring you to orgasm.

257. Milk the Penis

One of the fun benefits of having a toned PC muscle is that you'll have the ability to "milk" your partner's penis with your vagina—also known as *pompoir*. Once your partner is inside of you, what you'll want to do is begin clenching your PC muscle for 5 to 10 seconds at a time. Go up to 20 reps. As you do this, the sensation of wrapping your vagina around his penis may cause you to orgasm. But if you can manage to stave off your pleasure for just a moment, this clenching and releasing will make your partner feel as if you are "milking" his penis and it won't be long until his penis erupts, releasing a powerful orgasm.

258. Change Your Lifestyle

Do you smoke cigarettes or overindulge in alcohol and food? Kicking these unhealthy habits can have a real effect on the intensity of your orgasm. Smoking and being overweight can cause the blood vessels to shrink and this leads to a smaller amount of blood flowing to the penis and vulva—which means a less powerful orgasm.

In addition, for overweight or obese men in particular, losing weight will not only have an impact on the strength of your erection, you'll see yourself gain inches—that's right, inches—because you'll have less fatty tissues surrounding the base of your penis. How's that for motivation?

259. Boost Your Libido

It's unreasonable to expect yourself to be in the mood at any given moment, but if you've been struggling with finding your sex drive, here are some things you can do to improve your desire to pounce on your partner. For women, troubles in the bedroom are often tied to anxiety. Try to relax in the moment and not worry about everything else that needs to be done.

But if you believe that most of your problems stem from guilt, shame, fear of unfilled desire, or another emotional feeling that is holding you back, sometimes it's best to share these with your partner. If sharing doesn't alleviate your problem, it may be worth seeing a therapist to work through deeper issues.

260. Try Herbal Remedies for Extra Help

If you've ever browsed the shelves of a health food store or the vitamin aisle, you know there are many herbs available on the market that claim to have a positive impact on all sorts of ailments . . . including sexual prowess and desire. Before you decide to take any, do some research to make sure it doesn't conflict with any other medication you're currently taking (for instance, St. John's Wort is said to be an antidepressant, but it also makes birth control less effective). Here are some that claim to help with sexual issues.

- Ginkgo biloba: This herb increases the concentration of dopamine and other neurotransmitters that increase pleasure, happiness, and alertness. In doing so, it may also boost your sex drive and desire to bed your partner. Or the guy at the next table.
- Ginseng: This root increases the production of sex hormones and helps boost stamina. It also helps moderate stress and can reduce the symptoms of menopause.
- Avena sativa (wild oats): This plant produces deep relaxation, is said to increase sex drive, and creates stronger erections. It also may boost men's testosterone levels.

- Muira puama: Known as "potency wood," this unique plant heightens the physical response and sensations to sexual stimuli. It increases sex drive and intensifies erections and, so far, has no known harmful side effects. It's been used in Europe for centuries and is now slowly gaining popularity in the United States.
- Black cohosh: This herb is said to improve premenstrual symptoms as well as lubrication and sexual responsiveness in women because of its effects on the female hormones estrogen and progesterone.
- Dong quai: This herb relaxes menstrual cramps, supports and balances hormone production, and relaxes the smooth muscles in the body. It also has pain-relieving effects stronger than aspirin.
- Ashwagandha: This native plant of India stimulates the body to produce the precursors to testosterone and progesterone and can have a positive effect on sexual response and sex drive.

DID YOU KNOW?

As you've been reading throughout this book, taking care of yourself is not only important for your health, it can also increase your ability to orgasm tenfold. If you have been feeling stressed or rundown lately and your sex life has taken a serious hit, consider taking a day off of work and pampering yourself. Take a long, hot bath with your favorite salts or bubbles, get a massage, read your favorite book, listen to soft music, paint your nails, walk around your house naked, cook a delicious meal, watch your favorite romantic comedy film, explore a little self-love—anything that suits your fancy.

If you are too wound up to relax, try making your house a worry-free zone by meditating (you can find some great guided meditations on YouTube), or by creating a worry list. A worry list is a list of, well, your worries. But after every worry is listed, you have to write at least one viable and practical solution to resolve that worry. If you can't come up with a solution, perhaps it isn't something you should even worry about! For example, you might write, "I'm worried that I'm not fulfilling my duties at work," followed by, "I can have a check-in with my manager on Monday and ask if there is anything I can improve on." Sometimes having a workable solution to your worries makes them way easier to face.

If you truly spend your "you day" relaxing and taking care of yourself, the odds that you'll jump on your partner the second he comes home are much, much higher!

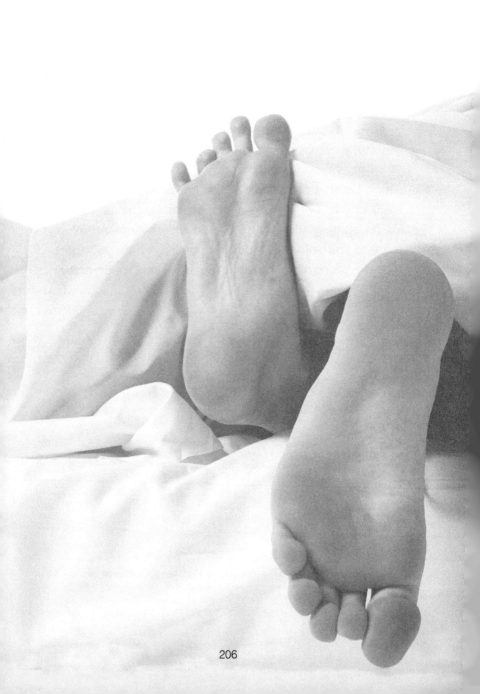

CHAPTER FOURTEEN

Location, Location, Location

261. Pick the Place

Having sex in the bedroom is great, but that's not the only place where you can get it on. And when you're looking for new locations, *where* you're going to have sex can be almost as critical to the moment as who you're with and what position you're in. For instance, if you're a voyeur, the sex might be heightened by watching yourself and your partner do it in front of a mirror. If you're an exhibitionist, your sexual escapades could be taken to the next level by discreetly—or not so discreetly—doing it in a public place where there is an actual risk of getting caught. But if exhibitionism freaks you out, then having sex in public would make it very difficult for you to reach orgasm. The next few tips explore some of the places outside of the bedroom where you might enjoy getting busy.

262. Have Sex in the Shower

Having sex in the shower can be a lot of fun. Whether you engage in oral sex, mutual masturbation, or penetrative sex, the shower is a great space for it. Begin by enticing your partner to shower with you, and, as you're washing each other, take the sensuality of that experience to the next level by washing and caressing his chest and penis. Ask him to return the favor. Once you've started to turn each other on and everything is getting fun and sudsy, you can go down on your partner so he can feel the dual sensation of your mouth on him as the water rushes over his body. Or, if you desire, you can skip more foreplay and move right on to sex. Having sex *can* be a bit tricky in the shower, as there's often limited space to move around in, and very little to brace yourself on. Standing and rear-entry positions, such as doggie style, often work best. If this idea turns you on at all, the next time you're at the store, pick up some of those nonslip adhesives to stick to the bottom of the tub so you and your partner don't keel over while you're having fun!

263. Get Dirty in the Bathtub

Though messing around in the tub is similar to hooking up in the shower, having sex in the bath offers a different sort of experience. If you're having sex in a Jacuzzi or a hot tub, you experience the fun of using the jets, which when focused on your clitoris or the head of a man's penis can lead to an orgasm all on their own! Or, if you're just having sex in a standard tub, the feeling of having the water sloshing around both of you has the power to arouse as you might know from the tips I provided on masturbating while bathing. Some positions that work well in a small tub include the fluttering butterfly or rear-entry positions that don't require either person to spread out for balance. Positions where you are sitting with your back against your partner can work in tight quarters as well.

264. Enjoy (Real) Sex on the Beach

Everyone claims they want to have sex on the beach. That is, until they start having sex on the beach. Then, they're more likely to spend most of the time groaning, not from pleasure but because they have sand in areas where they really didn't want it, such as inside their vagina. My suggestion? Dodge the sand problem altogether and do it in the ocean. If the water is warm, as it is in parts of Florida or the Bahamas, it will be easy for the man to become aroused and you two can enjoy the sensation not only of the surrounding water moving against you but also the fun of kissing underwater and feeling free in nature. The best positions for having sex in the water are, of course, those that involve standing. In fact, the water is a perfect place to try these out because while you can't brace yourself against a wall, the water gives you more buoyancy so even less buff partners will have an easier time keeping up their stamina in this position.

Of course, if you really want to try having sex on the shore à la *From Here to Eternity*, go for it. Just don't tell me I didn't warn you.

265. Be Outdoorsy

You don't have to be a hippie to have fun in the woods. If you can find a secluded hiking trail, picturesque forest, or another outdoor space that evokes your love of nature, why not bring your partner there for some loving? The different scents and visual stimuli can be a real turn-on for both of you. Think about it—wouldn't it be fun to have sex in the crunchy autumn leaves with the aroma of fall all around? Or in a quiet garden as flowers are blooming in the springtime? Or in the hushed darkness that comes just after the first snowfall? When you switch up your location, it's easier to create lasting memories that you can reflect back on and remember together.

266. Become a Member of the Mile-High Club

Though flight attendants pay more attention to how many people are in the bathroom at one time these days (which is how some celebrities have gotten caught in the act), this is a fun one to try if you can manage to not get caught. Of course, the rush of potentially getting in trouble is part of the fun. The best time to try this is if you find yourself on a mostly empty flight, or during a long overnight flight. If you do, and you can casually sneak off to the bathroom and have your partner join you, you'll probably get a rush out of the experience, though you might later get some dirty looks from the flight attendants even if they don't bust you.

Another alternative is booking a package with a hot air balloon company or a small airline service that offers a mile-high package. Though you won't get the rush from being a rebel, you will get the enjoyment of having sex in the air.

267. Get Off in Public

For real exhibitionists who get off on being caught, or at least being seen by others while you have sex, try masturbating your partner, giving head, or, if you're feeling really daring, actually having sex in public. If you don't want to be caught, wear a flowing skirt or dress that you can lift up enough in the back so that your partner can penetrate you while no one around is the wiser. A slightly less public option is to have sex in the back of a taxicab. Though you only have one potential audience member, it may do the trick for you. If you want to try this, tip the driver well ahead of time and climb on top of your beloved for your own ride.

268. Get Busy at the Office

When you're stuck at your office on a late night, you may have fantasized about how much more fun it would be to do it on your office desk than to send one more e-mail or put out one more fire. If you are sure that your company has no cameras that are taping what's going on behind your office door, invite your lover up late one night and live out your fantasy. It'll bring a smile to your face the next time you're stuck at the office working on an endless project.

269. Make Love in the Elevator

It can be a lot of fun to have sex in places you're not supposed to and in places you might get caught. One alternative to doing it in the office is to have sex in the elevator of an office building. Late at night, when there's no one around, pull the stop button in the elevator and have a quickie while you're hanging stories above the ground. Just do it fast enough that you don't incur the wrath of security or the fire department. If you're going to try that maneuver, I recommend not doing it at your own office, as someone is usually keeping an eye on what's going on inside those moving contraptions.

270. Put Your Orgasm Into Overdrive

If having sex in places other than inside your home appeals to you but you're not ready to make love outdoors or in public, try having sex in your car. You can do it in the front seat, in the backseat, or even on the roof! While on a road trip, get your partner in the mood by turning the conversation toward sex and then ramp things up by caressing their thigh and stomach as they—or you—drive. When you see a good spot to pull off the road—perhaps a country road that runs alongside the highway—exit, and get it on. Depending on the size of your car, it might be a bit tricky to find a good position, but rear-entry positions and those with the female on top work well even if you have a small car. For an extra rush, try doing it at a scenic overlook or at a drive-in movie theater.

271. Leave No Household Surface Unloved

Tired of having sex in bed but it's too cold outside to have sex comfortably outdoors? Then start finding new places to do it in your home. Have your lover bend you over the kitchen table. Try having sex on the floor. On the stairs. Over the arm of the couch. Really, wherever the mood takes you. Pretend you're teenagers again and get creative! Spots in your house that you usually wouldn't consider sexually appetizing may work great for set pieces. And, making a sexual connection with rooms around the house can also help boost your sex drive when you remember the fun times that happened there.

272. Bounce Along with the Spin Cycle

Doing laundry is dull, but the spin cycle, well, that can be a lot of fun. For both men and women, the vibrations the washing machine makes as it is wringing the water from your wet clothes can not only start the cycle of desire, they could cause you to have an orgasm. For a fun, intense experience, lean up against the washer during the spin cycle and have your partner take you from behind. The combination of your partner's thrusting and the vibrating of the machine will stimulate your G-spot and your clitoris at the same time.

273. Redecorate with Sex Wedges

If the furniture you have just isn't quite right for the sexual positions you're trying to achieve or you (or your partner) are not as flexible as you need to be, it's time to try a sex prop. On the market, there are ramps, wedges, cubes, and balls designed specifically for sex that can help you reach the position you're looking for and possibly discover some new ones in the process. Remember how in *Meet the Fockers*, Rozalin Focker's class carries around those foam cushion-like objects? Those are sex wedges. And as you might remember, they were quite large. In other words, you'll have to find a convenient place to store them before company comes unless you want to come up with a creative answer about where you got your unique new "couch."

274. Install a Love Swing

Even less discreet than sex wedges are love swings. These devices hang from the ceiling and allow you and your partner to try out positions that are impossible otherwise. The device is attached to the ceiling and has places to put your butt, arms, and legs so you can navigate yourself into pretty much any position you can imagine as you're suspended in the air. If you've been dreaming of having sex as part of a Cirque du Soleil production, this is definitely the toy for you.

DID YOU KNOW?

Even if they won't admit it, many people get a thrill out of knowing someone is watching them when they are naked or partially undressed and in a "private" moment. (Of course, this assumes that you are aware you are being watched and are okay with it. This is totally different from being the victim of a peeping Tom, which most people find disturbing and not the least bit sexy—not to mention illegal.)

As an exhibitionist, you are mainly enjoying the fact that you know the person (or people) watching you finds you and your activities sexy and exciting. You have his undivided attention, and he is totally captivated by your every move. You can get a strange sense of power by knowing you have this effect on someone else.

Remember, just because you like someone watching you in an intimate moment doesn't necessarily mean you want to have an intimate moment with him. Most exhibitionists like to keep their show a strictly one-sided performance. Some people who engage in a swinging or open lifestyle do take their exhibitionism to the next level and invite their audience to join in. But it's very possible to be an exhibitionist and still be in a faithful, monogamous relationship.

If you and your partner are interested in this, like all things, make sure you communicate your expectations and what you are comfortable with, including being recorded.

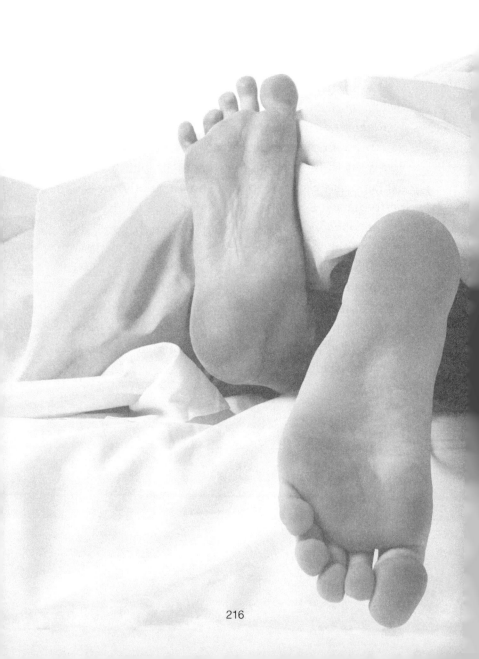

CHAPTER FIFTEEN

Perfect Your Sensual Bag of Tricks

275. Explore the Senses

You've experimented with different positions. You've tried out different places. Now, let me help you spice up your sex life with these sensual tips. One of the easiest ways to add some heat to the bedroom is by paying special attention to the senses. By temporarily removing at least one of the senses, the abilities of the others seem to strengthen to make up for their loss. For instance, if you have your partner shut his eyes, he will have to use his sense of smell, taste, touch, and hearing to understand the experience.

276. Use a Blindfold

Want your lover to ache with desire as they anticipate your next move in bed? Then use a blindfold or create your own using a scarf or silk sash. Ties can work as well in a pinch, but often they're too thin to really cover the eyes for the full effect. As you work your way over his body, ask him to keep the blindfold on, no matter how much he wants to remove it. This will build the sexual tension as your partner awaits your next move with nervous excitement and help intensify his eventual orgasm.

277. Tickle with Feathers

One way to tease your partner's senses is by using a feather wand. A feather wand is essentially a long pole with a few feathers on the end. These can be found at most sex stores, but you can improvise by using a new feather duster from the drugstore or even a cat toy.

Begin by tracing the feathers over his skin lightly and intersperse this light sensation with deep kisses and caresses. You'll soon have him quivering in excitement and enjoyment and his body will be primed for pleasure when you want to take it up a notch.

278. Warm Your Mouth with Hot Tea

Temperature is fun to use to activate the senses. Some people like the sensation of heat, while others prefer cold. If your lover is more of the warm variety, one way to pleasure him is to take a mug of just slightly warm tea and press it against his erogenous zones. Be careful not to spill any, as it may scald, but, especially if you do this on a chilly winter night, the warmth of the mug will send waves of pleasing sensations throughout your partner's body. Another way to use hot tea is by putting some in your mouth before you go down on him. Let the warm tea heat up your mouth, spit it out, and then begin to give him head. The warm temperature of your mouth will almost convince him that he's inside your vagina, so it's an especially good tactic to try when you're not able—or not in the mood—to have penetrative sex.

279. Heat Things Up with Wax

Another way to play around with heat is through the use of candles and hot wax. For your partner to enjoy this, he will likely have to have a reasonably high threshold for pain or for heat, as the initial sensation can be a bit intense. Take a just-extinguished candle—any candle will do though for the best effect, I wouldn't use anything smaller than a votive—and slowly pour the hot wax onto your partner. Start with a small, less sensitive area, as this will be less painful for him and it's a good way to test out whether or not he enjoys this. The feeling as the wax cools is an exciting one, and may leave your partner desiring more—more of you and more of the wax. Another option is to use a massage candle. These burn like regular candles, but the wax is made from an oil that, when liquid, can be used for massage, giving you two toys in one.

280. Cool It Down with Ice

If your lover is more the type to run out into the snow or the only person you know who actually *enjoys* cold showers, you may want to bring a little ice into the bedroom. Do this by cooling down sex toys you want to use on him—such as handcuffs—by submerging them in cold or icy water or by using actual ice cubes.

One fun thing to do is to take an ice cube and, starting at the top of your partner's chest or back, run it all the way down the body, holding it with your mouth if you can. The ice itself will bring the nerves to attention, and the runoff water from the ice will send tingles down your partner's spine. You can also try pressuring the erogenous zones with icy water (similar to what was done with the hot tea in Tip 278) to see if your partner likes that sensation.

281. Get Minty Fresh

Not only will mints temporarily improve your breath and make you that much more kissable, they're a fun and inexpensive little toy to use during oral sex. When you're about to go down on your partner, pop one in your mouth and start pleasuring him. The mint will cause a tingly sensation for your partner as you lick and suck down below that many people find extremely enjoyable. Have him return the favor when he's going down on you.

282. Try Gloves

Gloves aren't just for staying warm in the winter and looking fancy at night. They can also be for sexual play. Not only do they look sexy on their own, as they highlight the shape of the hands and arms, but you can also experiment with all of the different fabrics— leather, vinyl, rubber, silk, or even just plain old acrylic—to find out what sort of textures cause your lover to moan the most. To play with gloves in the bedroom, put them on when you're exploring your partner's erogenous zones. You may find that certain fabrics make your partner's skin come alive and have him doing his best not to pounce on you until you're done.

283. Spin the Wartenberg Wheel

This device looks a lot more frightening than it feels. With its steel handle and rotating wheel at the end covered in sharp spikes, it resembles a medieval torture device, but it's really a doctor's instrument designed to test the nerves. And yes, if you push too hard, it can be painful.

However, if your lover is the type who enjoys being scratched even just a little bit, pick up one of these and run it very lightly over your partner's skin. The tiny prickles felt from the device can feel extremely good and get those sexual fires burning, especially if you do him the pleasure of using it on his erogenous zones.

284. Pull Your Partner's Hair

Much earlier in Tip 19, you learned how the scalp is an erogenous zone. One way to activate the nerve endings there is by tugging on your partner's hair. To do this right, don't only pull on a few hairs at a time. That's a recipe for pain. Instead, be bold and grab a handful of his hair and slowly pull harder and harder until you release. Ask your partner if they liked that sensation and if they'd like for you to pull harder—or less hard—the next time.

Once you've learned where your partner's level is, some great times to try this are while you're kissing or while your partner is going down on you. By stimulating the erogenous zone of the scalp, you can get your partner going, too.

285. Whip Your Partner Into Shape

It doesn't take a professional dominatrix to wield a whip in the bedroom. It just takes some confidence. There are many types of whips, and some are more playful than others. The short ones that look like mini octopi don't really sting but provide the anticipation that can be a turn-on. Others, like the crop or full-on flogger/cat-o-nine-tails, are for those who enjoy a bit of stinging and can be used as hard or as soft as your partner would like. Experiment with different sensations. Try cracking the whip or crop on your partner for a quick sting, or just allow your partner to feel the sensation of having what can feel like multiple fingers touching him at once by drawing the toy over his body . . . perhaps before giving him some lashes.

286. Get Naughty with a Spanking

While getting spanked as a kid wasn't much fun, being spanked as an adult can be a turn-on. Test the waters to see if your partner enjoys the feeling of being spanked by giving them a nice firm whack on the butt during sex, then rubbing the area. For newcomers to the practice, here's a tip: *Always rub.* It dissipates the stinging sensation and replaces it with one of pure pleasure. If you discover that this is something your partner really enjoys, consider buying a paddle or have your partner lean over your legs or get on all fours while you give him a few good hard spanks.

287. Apply Liquid Latex

If your lover enjoys the pulling sensation that occurs when you remove the hot wax from Tip 279 off of his body, you may want to try using some liquid latex in the bedroom. You can use it to paint your lover in attractive colors, then gently pull it off after the latex has dried. But unless you're planning to cause pain, make sure to coat the body with a layer of lotion first. Also, unless your partner is aroused by the feeling of pain—and some people are—avoid the genitals. The pulling sensation there would be extremely painful. Before you pull it off, add a bit of liquid latex polish (also available at the sex store) so you and he can easily glide over each other and have some fun gliding together.

288. Try a Sex Toy

Though the human body is capable of delivering a lot of pleasure to another, sometimes it's fun to experiment with toys that do things our bodies cannot . . . such as vibrate extremely quickly. That's where sex toys come in.

There are many types of sex toys, from those that go inside to those that stay outside to those that do both. Some vibrate while others don't. In the tips that follow you'll find out all about the different types of sex toys. One thing to keep in mind about them: Don't share. Sharing sex toys is a good way to pass bacteria and even diseases. But if you must share, use your sex toy with a condom.

289. Try a Penetrating Sex Toy

For a change of pace, try bringing a dildo or vibrator—the most common penetrating toys—into the bedroom. You can use them to masturbate your partner, or you can watch your partner masturbate with them (after which, you might find yourself quite turned on). Or you can add them to your usual sex play and use them in place of—or in addition to—his penis in any of the positions and manual stimulation techniques I've already mentioned or any from your own library of favorites.

290. Do It with a Dildo

Dildos are a great entry into the world of penetrative sex toys. For the most part, most of them resemble a male penis and don't have any vibrating parts you have to adjust to your liking while you're penetrating yourself with them. In other words, using a dildo is pretty straightforward—just stick it in . . . after you're aroused, of course.

Dildos can vary in size, shape, and appearance and come with or without testicles. Some are ridged while others are smooth, and some might, like artificial vaginas for men, be cast from the penises of male adult stars. They can also come in a range of the following materials:

- PVC or jelly—These dildos are usually the least expensive. There's a reason why. They're porous, which means that if you use them without a condom, bacteria can lurk in their surfaces and give you a dangerous infection. Plus, some cheaper ones may release cancer-causing phthalates. Save your money and spring for silicone.
- Silicone—These dildos have replaced the PVC and jelly dildos as the standard go-to dildo. As they're a bit more rigid than the PVC dildo, they feel more similar to a male penis. Plus, they don't have a plastic smell and they hold body heat, so if you plan on using these for years, they're a better choice. They can be cleaned easily and sterilized by immersing them in boiling water.
- Glass or metal—These dildos are very rigid and can be used to practice Kegel exercises or incorporated into temperature play, as they conduct both heat and cold very well. They are easy to clean but they're also the most expensive, as they are more expensive to construct.

291. Try a G-Spot Dildo

Your G-spot doesn't have to be stimulated with just your fingers or by a partner. There are many toys on the market that will help you stimulate this sometimes hard-to-find spot within your vagina. The toys that do this have a unique, almost banana-like shape to them, and can be used just like a dildo, but they're built specifically to stimulate your G-spot. To find them, look for the extremely curved dildos that resemble a C in the sex shop.

292. Give It a Go with a Vibrator

Once you've gotten the hang of how to use a dildo to reach orgasm or get yourself awfully close, why not try a vibrator? Vibrators, which run on electric or battery power, are often small, discreet, and external, and are designed to stimulate the clitoris and other parts of the vulva. However, others, like the infamous Rabbit, have a vibrating portion designed to stimulate the clitoris and another dildo-like portion that can be inserted to stimulate the vagina with the moving beads within its shaft. When you first start masturbating using a vibrator, begin at a low speed and then work your way up. You may even consider trying it out on your inner thigh or stomach first to get the hang of it before directly stimulating your vulva.

293. Experiment with Dual-Action Dildos

Not all vibrators and dildos on the market are intended solely for women. Some are meant to work for couples. Those designed for male-female or male-male couples have a ring that is meant to go around your partner's penis and an attached vibrating bullet that can stimulate your clitoris or his perineum.

Others, such as double-ended dildos, have penile tips on both ends that can be used either to stimulate one woman vaginally and anally or two women at the same time. If you and your partner are new to the world of dual-pleasure vibrators or dildos, I recommend shopping for one together so you can find a toy that you both want to try.

294. Use Household Objects

Just because you want to play around with sex toys doesn't mean you have to buy them from the store. For women, dry humping a pillow or other soft but structured objects can stimulate the clitoris, and I'm sure you can think of plenty of foods that could be used in place of a dildo. And for men, just use your imagination to come up with something that he could penetrate. A melon, perhaps? Get creative!

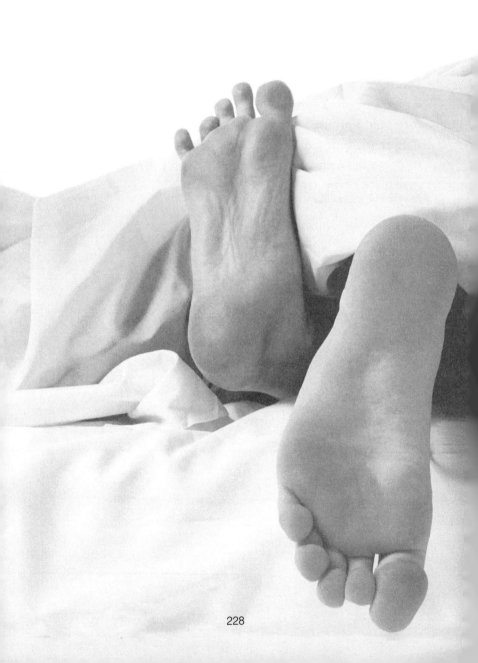

CHAPTER SIXTEEN

All Tied Up with No Place to Go . . .

295. Play with Restraint

Curious about what it's like to be all tied up and have nowhere to go after reading *Fifty Shades of Grey*? Want to create your own Red Room? Being physically restrained in bed for pleasure requires a lot of trust, but succumbing to your partner can be a liberating experience. When your partner ties you up or binds your hands so that you can't prevent your partner from arousing you, you'll find your whole body becomes a lightning rod for pleasure as you try and move the parts of yourself that you want touched toward your partner's mouth or hands. The next few tips will cover some of the most basic ways to restrain your partner as well as other popular toys used by the BDSM community.

296. Cuff 'Em

The most common type of restraint are handcuffs. Handcuffs come in a variety of types, from plastic ones that break easily to fake fur–covered metal ones you can unlock without a key to nearly official police handcuffs that not even Houdini could have found his way out of. Okay, well, maybe Houdini could have, but you can't. If your lover doesn't enjoy the metal against his skin (as handcuffs can dig into the flesh), swap out handcuffs for restraint tape or silk rope. These can also be used to restrain your partner, but they don't cause the same amount of friction on the skin.

When your partner is tied up, have fun teasing them—and perhaps employing some of the tips I suggested earlier such as the hot wax, ice, feathers, or other ways to activate his senses. By the time you begin touching his genitals, he'll be begging for release . . . and it's up to you to decide when you want to give it to him.

297. Put a Ring on It

Cock rings—usually made from leather, metal, or rubber—are devices that are placed around the base of the penis or around both testicles and the base of the penis in order to help the wearer maintain a firmer, longer-lasting erection by reducing the blood flow out of the penis's erectile tissue. Until you get a handle on how much pressure he can take, I recommend starting with the leather or rubber type, as you could cut these off if the sensation becomes too great. Once you have learned the size of cock ring that works best for you, feel free to try the metal variety. But don't use them when you're using a pill like Viagra, and don't leave one on for more than a half hour, as they can cause nerve damage if he's wearing them for an extended period of time.

298. Spread the Balls

Ball spreaders are a type of cock ring that also lift and separate the testicles or stretch the scrotum. Unlike cock rings, which are mostly for functional use or aesthetic appeal, these devices gently pull, stretch, and tease the testicles, and some include weights that create a heavier pulling sensation. Some men find these to be very pleasurable and discover that they intensify their orgasm.

299. Silence Your Partner with a Ball Gag

Ball gags are devices that feature a strap that goes around the head and a device that goes in the mouth. The portion that goes into the mouth is typically ball-shaped, though it can also be shaped like a penis to offer the sensation of double penetration if the gag is used during sex. When used in tandem with other restraint devices, these can heighten the anticipation and desire of both parties, as it becomes a nonverbal game when the one restrained craves release and the one doing the restraining has to decide how—and when—they want that to happen.

Don't have a ball gag handy but you or your partner want to experience the feeling of what one would be like? Use a handkerchief, scarf, or another item that can be tied around the head and inserted into the mouth instead. Just be careful not to insert too much fabric into the mouth, as you don't want to cause accidental choking.

300. Clamp It Down with Nipple Clamps

Nipples can be very sensitive erogenous zones for both men and women, and some people enjoy the feeling of their nipples being pinched or bitten. If you or your partner is into this type of play, clamps are one possible next step. Nipple clamps are essentially modified clothespins and when attached, cause pain and intense pressure for the wearer that your lover may find pleasurable. Try using them when you're also doing something to your partner that you know they'll love—such as going down on them—so they can experience both pleasure and pain in the same moment.

301. Be Dominant

Engaging in power play can be a lot of fun for a couple, especially if the roles of who is in charge are switched from what the norm is for the two of you. When trying out the dominant role, tell your partner that he has to do whatever you ask in bed, and command him to lick, touch, and kiss you in all the places you desire.

You may find that your partner really enjoys pleasing you as you guide him around your body. Some couples like to take this a step further and start a master/slave relationship where the master controls all aspects of the slave's life, and some even extend this far outside the bedroom.

302. Be Submissive

If you're used to controlling the action, take a step back for a change. Tell your partner you'll do anything they ask of you in the bedroom. As you pleasure him, you may feel a deeper connection as you learn what your partner enjoys, and you can use this knowledge in your next "free play" session of sex.

303. Use Safe Words

When you're engaging in dominant and submissive behavior or restraint play, it's worth it to designate a safe word. Because this is the only type of play during which "no" and "stop" can actually mean "yes," if you really don't want to do something or want your partner to stop, using the word "no" can be ineffective. Pick a word you'll remember and one you likely wouldn't typically use during sex. This way when your partner moans "No," you know that you can keep going with their consent, but if they say "Hamster!," then you need to stop what you're doing and make sure they're okay.

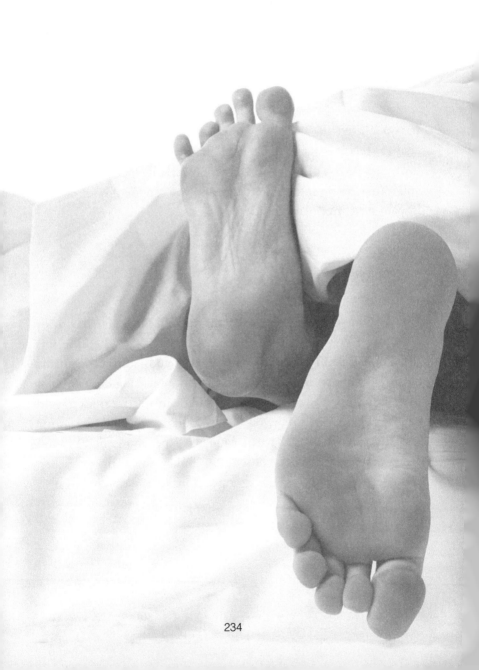

CHAPTER SEVENTEEN

Unleash Your Kinky Side

304. Try Something a Little More Kinky

If you've tried restraints, power play, and tactile sensation toys, it might be time to add something a little more intense to kick your sex life into an even kinkier territory. The next few tips will cover some sexual behaviors and objects that are a little more out of the ordinary, from penis pumps to lactation play. But as I've said before, if both parties are up for the experience, anything goes!

305. Pump It Up

Penis pumps, which often resemble a giant vacuum tube, are used to manually pump blood into the erectile tissue and create a larger, firmer erection either for the partner to gaze at or for functionality if someone has a hard time becoming erect (in which case, using one may help him reach a more satisfying orgasm). They work by using suction but can only help maintain an erection temporarily, so if you're looking to keep the penis as hard as you've made it using the pump, you need to place a cock ring on as well to block the blood flowing back into the body.

306. Use a Clitoris or Vaginal Pump

Clitoral and vaginal pumps are similar to the penis pump except that there is no real need to use them for the purpose of penetration. These pumps are mostly for aesthetic pleasure as some people find it arousing to gaze at a particularly swollen clitoris or vagina. However, some fans of these pumps have reported that they can increase the intensity of orgasm. Some pumps also have vibrating features, but some women find that sensation a bit too intense. So if you're considering trying one, I recommend starting out with the basic pump first and working your way up to a more high-tech device.

307. Swell Your Nipples

In addition to penis and clitoral pumps, there are also nipple pumps. These can be used on men or women to enlarge the nipples to a swollen state where they are extremely sensitive, and some may find them pleasurable to gaze upon. To plump up the nipples, you can use a snakebite kit from a camping store, suction cups, or vacuum pumps, but be careful not to overdo it, as you can cause damage to the nerves or tissue by using these devices too often.

308. Add to the Fun with Penis Extenders

If you want to penetrate your partner more deeply or, to reach orgasm, you want to be penetrated farther than your partner is physically able to do, no matter what the position, consider a penis extender or sleeve. This hollow device attaches directly to the penis to increase its length or girth and is made from a variety of materials, from Cyberskin to silicone.

309. Tickle Her Pink with a French Tickler

Though some people regard these as merely novelty condoms, French ticklers are condoms with different types of protrusions on the end. Some are nubby, others are hair-like, and others also serve as penis extenders. Using them can cause the person being penetrated to feel sensations that a regular penis can't deliver, so because of that I like to think of them like the different attachments for a screwdriver. And the different protrusions can stimulate your vagina in different ways—and possibly help your partner reach those tricky areas such as the A-spot. After all, while there's nothing wrong with the original, standard penis, sometimes it's fun to have a little variety!

310. Get Into High-Tech Sex

We know there's electricity between you and your partner, but what about creating some real sparks? In erotic electrostimulation you stimulate the body's nerves with low-frequency sensations via a power source, such as a Violet wand, in order to bring pleasure. If you choose to engage in this type of stimulation, do so very carefully, as even low voltages can cause permanent damage. Because of this, I am not going to go into detail on how to use these devices in this book, as I'd rather you receive a more thorough explanation in person from the knowledgeable clerk at your local sex shop.

311. Milk It for All It's Worth

For some men and women, the sight of breasts heavy with milk can turn them on, as can watching a woman squeeze milk from her full breasts. Sometimes this fetish begins when a couple has their first child, but with some people it begins even earlier, and it has been found that, given the right amount of hormones and stimulation, it is possible for women to start producing milk again or for women who have never had children to produce milk to satisfy themselves and their partners.

312. Puncture for Pleasure: Genital Piercings

Over the last two decades, piercings have become no longer counterculture, but genital piercings are still considered to be relatively taboo. However, those with them often find that they can help cause more intense orgasms when they're fondled during sexual play or that, because of their placement, having these areas stimulated throughout the day can be very pleasant. Here are a few of the most common:

- Prince Albert: This piercing runs through the outside of the frenulum and up and out through the urethra of the penis or a hole created in the glans.
- Clitoral hood piercing: This is the most common genital piercing for women, perhaps because the ring is able to easily stimulate the clitoris during sexual activity or when something a woman is wearing rubs up against it.
- Clitoris piercing: Less common than the clitoral hood piercing, this is said to cause immense sexual satisfaction, though there is a risk of injuring the nerves in the clitoris.
- Nipples: If the nipples of a man or woman are pierced properly, piercing them can awaken the nerves so that they are even more sensitive.

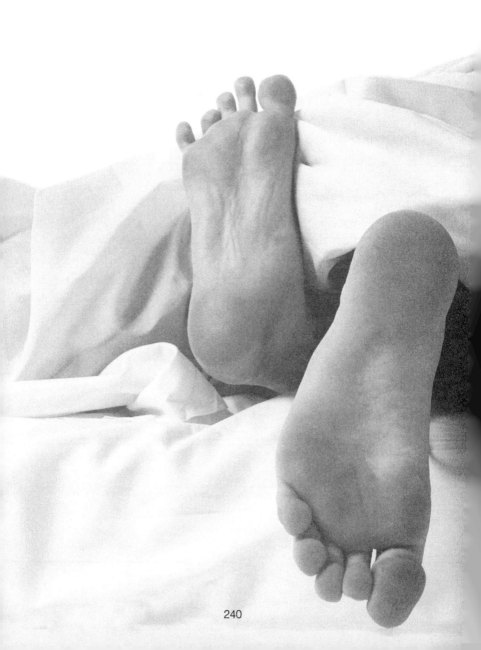

CHAPTER EIGHTEEN

Try the Back Door

313. Attempt Anal Penetration

For some, anal penetration is the final frontier, the orifice that must be avoided at all costs, while for others it's just another way to have sex. Whether you're thinking about trying anal sex for the first time or this is old hat to you, the following tips should provide you with some of the basics to help you enjoy anal sex as much as possible and to give those who love it some new techniques to try out. If you're hesitant about anal sex, consider that because the wall between the rectum and the vagina is very thin, anal sex can stimulate some of the more difficult-to-reach zones within the vagina (like the A-spot), at the same time leaving the vagina open for other play with fingers, tongues, or sex toys.

As with vaginal penetration, you can penetrate the anus with a penis, finger or fingers, or an inanimate object. But however you're penetrating the cavity and inching in past the sensitive opening, you will need much more lubrication than you think is necessary. That is because that part of the body does not release any natural lubrication. In addition, the sphincter muscle holding that part of the body closed requires a lot of lubricated massage to relax and be ready for penetration. And, as the skin here is very easy to tear, it is very important to engage in safe, well-lubricated sex when stimulating the anus.

In closing, ladies, as you and your partner enjoy having anal sex, make sure to switch condoms between anal and vaginal sex so that you don't pass bacteria. If you're not using protection, be sure to thoroughly wash any object that has been in the anus before using it to penetrate the mouth or vagina.

314. Don't Be a Tight Ass

Once you're ready and interested in having anal sex, you need to prepare your body for the experience. Anal sex, unlike vaginal sex, is not usually something that's possible to have as a quickie. The most important thing you can do—in addition to having a lot of silicone-based lubricant on hand—is to relax. And if you're not used to relaxing your anus (and more than likely, you're not), this will likely take some time. Begin by breathing deeply and trying to relax your body. Once you're at ease, have your partner begin to massage your anus and the surrounding area using the lubricant. When you're feeling fully relaxed and you don't feel like you are still clenching your anus, that's when you should move on to the next tip.

315. Try Finger Play

Earlier in this book, I provided a brief overview of how to stimulate a man's prostate gland by penetrating his anus (Tip 197). If you're a woman who wants to have anal sex, the technique your partner should use is the same. Either way, if the partner being penetrated is new to anal stimulation, I recommend going slowly. Very slowly. Your partner should make sure that their nails are trimmed and don't have any sharp edges while you enjoy a bath or shower. If it makes you feel more comfortable, you can douche anally or give yourself an enema. While douching is not recommended for the vagina, as it disrupts the delicate balance of the vagina's natural bacteria, it's fine for the rectum as long as you're gentle.

Then, once you're back in bed, you can start by messing around and making out in bed, or have your partner massage you and slowly work his way toward your anus. When your partner senses that you're relaxed enough for him to touch your anus—thanks to the deep breathing you were practicing in the last tip—he should add some lubrication to his finger and touch your anus using slow, circular motions, keeping the fleshy part of his finger perpendicular to the anal opening.

As he continues to add more lubrication and massage the anus, he should slowly increase the pressure, until he reaches the point when he finally feels the muscle relax. This is when he should slowly penetrate your anus with his finger and begin to explore inside.

316. Start Out with Anal Toys

Before jumping into full-on anal sex that involves a penis or dildo, try having your partner penetrate your anus using a smaller penetrative device, such as anal beads or a probe, so you can adjust to the sensation of having something go into your anus (versus out). Just as your partner did when he penetrated your anus with his finger, he should have patience when getting ready to penetrate you with a slightly larger object. One word of caution—don't fully insert anything without a serious handle into the anus. Unlike with the vagina, toys can actually get stuck in the rectum, and nothing's a bigger buzzkill than a trip to the emergency room.

317. Try a Butt Plug

Though they do have a terribly off-putting name (we dare you to try and say it romantically!), these sex toys can be inserted into the anus and can provide the rectum with a pleasurable sense of full-ness that can cause a strong orgasm in the person being penetrated. Their unique design—they are typically very narrow at the top and bottom with a wider middle section and a flattened bottom—also prevents them from being sucked up into the rectum. Though the basic butt plug is sleek and immobile, you can find ridged and vibrating plugs, and some are even capable of being inflated as large as the receiver desires.

318. Check Out Anal Beads

Like butt plugs, anal beads are inserted into the rectum to provide stimulation to the anus, but the sensation they deliver is a bit dif-ferent. These toys are composed of round, smooth beads strung together on a nylon, silicone, or cotton cord that is then lubricated and inserted into the anus before your partner is close to orgasm. When your partner senses that you are getting close to reaching orgasm—perhaps through both anal and vaginal or anal and cli-toral stimulation—they should gently tug on the string to pull out one bead at a time to intensify your orgasm.

If you're using a nylon or silicone cord, these can be cleaned and reused, but if you're using cotton, you need to use a different string each time to prevent the spread of bacteria.

319. Try Anal Probes

Once you're done cracking your alien abduction jokes, and you've already tried the anal toys suggested in the previous tips, it may be time to attempt the anal probe. This slender toy is shaped much like a penis's shaft and has a ball-like shape on the end. It will allow your partner to penetrate your anus deeper than he could with the butt plug or anal beads and it can help prepare you more fully for anal sex, as the device resembles his penis.

Like with butt plugs, anal probes come in many variations—including vibrating and beaded probes that function similarly to anal beads—and if you're using it on him, do note that if you move the anal probe in certain directions, it makes it easy to stimulate his prostate gland.

320. Stimulate His Prostate with a Toy

Most of the following tips have been centered around the idea that your partner will be penetrating you, but if he's the one who loves having his prostrate stimulated, consider picking up a device specifically made for doing just that. Like the dildos on the market specifically designed for stimulating your G-spot, there is also a toy for men—the prostate stimulator—that will stimulate his G-spot. These toys are angled in such a way that when inserted into the anus, they put a pleasurable amount of pressure both on the prostate and externally on the perineum so that you can stimulate the gland from both sides and bring him to a body-shaking, explosive orgasm.

321. Rim Your Partner

Analingus, also known as rimming, involves using your tongue or mouth to stimulate your lover's anus much in a similar way as a man would go down on a woman during cunnilingus. Because the anus is packed with nerves, this can be a very pleasurable sensation and a good lead-in to anal sex. However, rimming does require some precautions against bacteria and other diseases. First, have your partner shower and thoroughly wash his or her anus before pleasuring them. If it makes you (or your partner) feel more comfortable, stimulate him or her through a dental dam or a small piece of plastic wrap. To really turn on your partner using analingus, encircle the rim of the anus with your tongue, lick it from one side to the other, and even consider penetrating the anus with your tongue.

322. Go Slowly with Anal Sex

After your partner has warmed up your anus and you've become accustomed to the feeling of having something in your anus—you might be ready for anal sex. Make sure he uses a lot of silicone-based lubricant on both the condom and on your anus prior to entry and that he knows not to be shy about adding more during sex. Have him go slowly and gently, only gaining speed and adding pressure when you ask him to. The same goes for you if you're penetrating him with either an anal probe, dildo, or a strap-on. While he's penetrating you, if just the sensation of having anal sex isn't enough to bring you to orgasm, you can heighten the sensation and bring yourself closer to coming by stimulating your clitoris or playing with your vaginal opening.

323. Return to the Missionary Position

A big component to having great anal sex is the position. Whereas with vaginal sex, in which you may find that certain positions work better than others to help you reach orgasm, with anal sex you're most likely to discover that some positions feel good and some positions make you want to stop having anal sex immediately. The following two positions are great for anal sex, especially if you're new to the experience.

The first is the missionary. Having anal sex in the missionary position is essentially like having vaginal sex in this position. It's a great starting position because the rectum is straight and having sex puts very little pressure on its walls. Plus, it allows you and your partner to look at one another as you see if you both like this new addition to your sexual toolbox. Once you're comfortable with having anal sex in that position, you can vary it slightly by putting your knees up and having your partner kneel between them as he penetrates you.

324. Do It Doggie Style

When you think of anal sex, this is probably the position that comes to mind. But I don't recommend it for your first anal sex experience. That's because it doesn't give you much control. Also, because of the angle your bodies are at, his penis puts quite a bit of pressure on the walls of your rectum. While this pressure feels great during vaginal sex, it's probably going to be a while before this feels good for you during anal sex. However, once you're comfortable with having anal sex, this position is great for deep penetration, or if you're penetrating him, for prostate stimulation.

DID YOU KNOW?

In addition to adult movies, there is also the old-school type of pornography: magazines and pictures. These can be a way to become comfortable with adult images and ease your way into the material before you check out some X-rated films. Just as with films, these types of materials run the gamut from tame to wild. Again, it's a good idea to check out a few different types to find the styles that you and your partner like best.

For many couples, adult materials can be a great way to enhance their sex lives and bring some added excitement to the bedroom. But occasionally these materials can cause problems for one or both members of a couple. Some red flags:

- If you and/or your partner find it impossible to become aroused without the use of adult materials
- If one of you begins hiding your adult materials and covertly using them behind the other's back
- If one of you starts spending so much time viewing porn that your real-life sex life as a couple suffers

If any of these or other porn-related problems becomes an issue for you, it's probably time for you and your partner to have a serious discussion about porn's role in your relationship. Similarly, if the only times that your partner is interested in sex are prompted by adult materials or extreme experiences, you need to have a chat. In extreme cases, it might be necessary to enlist the help of a therapist or counselor.

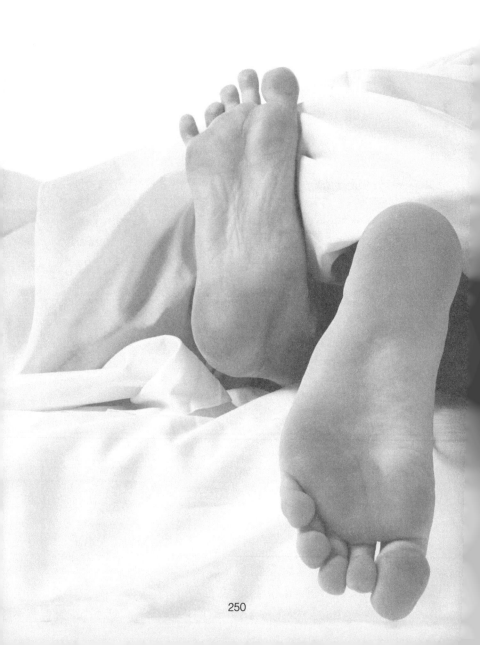

CHAPTER NINETEEN

Invite Some Company Over

325. Double Your Pleasure

For some women, the feeling of being penetrated by two penises at once can bring them to an almost instantaneous orgasm. But you don't have to have a threesome to make this happen. You and your partner alone can stimulate both your vagina and your anus. For instance, while you're having vaginal sex, he can insert a finger or toy into your anus—or vice versa—to give you that "full" sensation.

If you do want to try it in a threesome, this kind of sex can lead to an incredible orgasm for all parties. For you, it will provide the feeling of being "full" that can be arousing and orgasm-inducing on its own, and for the men, it allows them to both be stimulated not only by the vaginal or anal sex alone, but also by feeling the thrusting of the other man through the thin membrane that separates the vagina and the rectum. Just remember, if the guys are going to switch positions, have them put on new condoms.

326. Add a Third Wheel

Whether or not you want to try anal sex, adding another partner may be a way to add a spark to your sex life. For some, polyamory is a way of life. Unlike an affair, in the healthiest versions of these relationships, those involved enjoy having at least one steady partner and possibly one rotating sexual partner at a time with everyone's full knowledge and consent. But in the tips that follow, you'll find out how you can engage in polyamory while maintaining a primarily monogamous relationship.

327. Try a Threesome

Threesomes occur when three people get together for sexual play. The combination may involve two women and one man, two men and one woman, or three men or three women. The choice is up to you, your partner, and your combined sexual preferences. Sometimes the desire for a threesome arises out of one partner's desire to experiment with the opposite sex, or if a partner is bisexual, to have his or her sexual needs met by someone of the same sex.

To have a successful threesome, it's important to pay attention to the needs of your partner and set some ground rules you've discussed before beginning. Will there be penetration? What kind is okay? Is kissing okay between the new person and both partners? After sex, should the third party go home or should they sleep over? Should the threesome happen inside the home or at a neutral location like a hotel? Addressing these questions *before* finding or inviting a third party to join in will help prevent uncomfortable situations or hurt feelings afterwards. After your threesome, talk about how you feel about the experience. And be honest. You may find that it's something that you want to do more regularly or you may discover that it's caused issues that need to be resolved to rise to the surface.

BE HONEST

Threesomes can be a fun way to spice up your sex life, but they can also be a quick way to ruin your relationship if both parties are not secure and fully on board. Be honest with your partner if you don't want to do it, and encourage your partner to be honest about his feelings, too. Never agree to something just to make your partner happy, and make sure your partner does the same.

328. Play the Cuckold

One unique type of threesome involves three people in a room, but it typically involves you getting hot and heavy with a third party instead of with your partner. In cuckolding, a man watches his wife or girlfriend be penetrated or pleasured by another man, often someone who is bigger or more sexually capable than he is, while he watches and masturbates. The man who is in the relationship is known as the cuckold, the woman as the hot wife, and the third party as the bull. And while it may seem counterintuitive, the introduction of this new lover may draw the couple closer together, as the new person can cause the brain to release the neurochemicals of new love or attraction.

329. Be a Swinger, Baby

If you've tried a couple threesomes or foursomes and you and your partner find they do wonders for your sex life, you may want to take things to the next level by becoming a swinger and finding a couple (or couples) that you can swap partners with for the night. Though this type of swinging can happen spontaneously, if you're interested in checking out the lifestyle, do a little Internet research and start messaging those who seem in the know on polyamory-focused message boards. Strike up a friendship with one of those people and they may help you be able to find a swingers club in your area where you'll be able to meet other couples who are open to the experience. While no penetration usually occurs at these *Eyes Wide Shut*-esque parties, pretty much anything else goes. It's typically only at the on-premises, invite-only, prescreened parties where penetration happens, and where no alcohol is permitted.

330. Have an Accidental Orgy

Can't find a party? Throw one of your own. Though sex parties and orgies—sexual activity that occurs between more than three people—are often organized by local swinging clubs, you can encourage one to happen naturally if there's a lot of sexual tension in the air. It can start innocently with a game of Kings, Truth or Dare, or even Spin the Bottle, and then progress into something much more sexual.

331. Throw a Key Party

Or, if you have friends who you know are open to the idea of such a thing, throw a "key party." At these parties, all of the first guests who arrive put on a necklace with a lock on it, and then each new guest who comes to the party removes a key out of a bowl or hat. Each key corresponds to one of the locks and that's the person that they'll be partnered with, at least at the beginning of the night. Once passions start heating up, you never know what sort of swapping might happen.

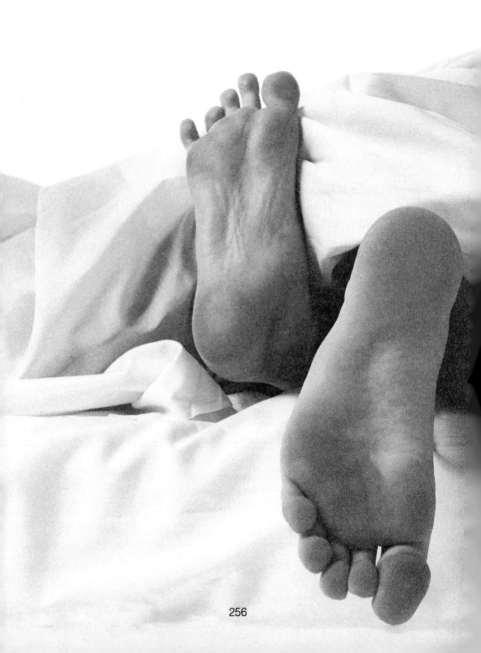

CHAPTER TWENTY

Embrace the Spiritual Side of Orgasms

332. Learn the Spiritual Side of Sex

Especially when you're with a loving partner, sex becomes more than just a physical act—it has a mental component as well. But did you know that there is also a spiritual side to sex? By engaging in a more spiritual type of sex—one that places more emphasis on the connection between you and your partner instead of orgasm, you might have some of the best orgasms of your life.

333. Discover the World of Tantra

Tantra is a Sanskrit word that can be roughly translated to mean "woven together" or "to expand." It is an ancient collection of beliefs that gained popularity in India between the eighth and twelfth centuries. The main tenet of the philosophy is that all things in our world are sacred, and followers of Tantra work to establish a spiritual connection with everything and everyone around them. They believe that by joining two seemingly opposite forces—the male and female, the dark and light, the hot and cold—this unity can lead to higher consciousness, joy, and enlightenment. And for you? A better orgasm.

334. Try Tantric Sex

Sex is just one part of the Tantric puzzle, but for the purpose of this book, it's the one we'll be focusing on. And, while I'll go into the basics of Tantric sex over the next few tips, if you really want to learn more about this subject in depth, I recommend the books *Introduction to Tantra: The Transformation of Desire* and *The Heart of Tantric Sex: A Unique Guide to Love and Sexual Fulfillment*.

What we know as tantric sex today stems from the newer (Neo Tantra) beliefs that put sex at the center, though both Tantra and Neo Tantra see desire as a step to spiritual awakening. In the older concept of Tantric sex, the focus is more on complete body happiness, experiencing expansive orgasms that do not necessarily include ejaculation, and finding ways to increase intimacy between you and your partner. The practice may also include activating the chakras and worshiping female energy.

335. Be Open to the Experience

Having a rewarding life (not to mention a great sex life) involves being open to new experiences and exploring avenues despite your skepticism. For instance, you may have some favorite foods that you were originally hesitant to try! The same goes for your sex life and Tantra. Even if you are mainly interested in tantric sex because of what you've heard about its ability to help you have profoundly intense orgasms, and you're skeptical about its spiritual side, take a chance and dive in fully to the practice. You may discover that it helps you develop a deeper connection with your partner, and as a result your relationship, sex life, and general quality of life may improve dramatically!

336. Understand Your Chakras

Those who follow the practice of Tantra believe that there are seven important centers, known as chakras, that run along your spine. The energy that flows through these and up the spine is known as kundalini energy. Each of these chakras corresponds to a different aspect of your spiritual being, and by releasing the blocked energy and balancing your chakras, Tantra's practioners believe you will be able to get that part of your body or spirit working.

If you've been having a difficult time achieving orgasm, Tantra's believers would suggest that you work on opening or balancing your first, second, and third chakras.

Chakra Number	Chakra Name	Location	Element	Color	Association
The First (Root) Chakra	Muladhara	Perineum	Earth	Red	Confidence, a realistic concept of our body and its needs, security and grounding in the physical comforts of life
The Second (Sacral) Chakra	Svad-hishthana	Genitals	Water	Orange	Pleasure, sexuality, stable emotions, gracefulness, self-acceptance, creativity
The Third (Navel) Chakra	Manipura	Solar plexus/navel	Fire	Yellow	Ego, self-esteem, energy, authority, longevity, reliability, independence
The Fourth (Heart) Chakra	Anahata	Heart	Air	Green	Sharing, love, service, compassion, devotion
The Fifth (Throat) Chakra	Vishuddha	Throat	Space	Violet	Truth, knowledge gained from other chakras
The Sixth (Third Eye) Chakra	Ajna	Pineal gland/third eye	None	Bluish-white	Enlightenment, self-realization, self-mastery, intuition, insight
The Seventh (Crown) Chakra	Sahasrara	Fontanel/top of the head	Lotus flower	Golden-white light	Supreme consciousness, compassion, self-awareness, mindfulness, awareness of the world

337. Open Your Chakras

Are you feeling "stuck" somewhere in your life? Feeling heartache? Headaches? Trouble fully releasing during orgasm? To become unstuck, you can use Tantra hand movements, or mudras, for some spiritual Drano. Each chakra has its own mudra position that helps open it. To help you get sexually unstuck, here are the positions for the first two chakras. If you're having difficulty in other areas, I encourage you to delve into deeper research on your own so you can heal them.

It's important to open and balance all chakras, but the most important chakra to work with might be the Root chakra. This is the chakra that grounds you, and it can be strengthened by physical activity and by holding the tip of your thumb and your index finger together. Concentrate as you do so on the sound "Lum."

The Sacral chakra holds the key to your sexual power, and you can open this one by placing your hands—left one on top of the right one—in your lap with the palms facing up with the tips of your thumbs gently touching. Concentrate as you do so on the sound "Vam."

Another way you can release your chakras is by having your partner give you a chakra massage. Lie on your back and, beginning at your lowest chakra, have your partner massage each chakra for several minutes until he has worked his way all the way up to the Seventh Chakra.

338. Know Your Tantric Vocabulary

As much as I would love to fully immerse you in the world of Tantra, there isn't the space in this book for a complete vocabulary lesson. But below, I've included some of the words that you'll need to know as we move forward and I teach you the basics of how to have mind-blowing orgasms through Tantric sex.

- Amrita—the female ejaculatory fluid that is considered a desirable life force in Tantra. (Tell that to your partner if he's shy about going down on you.)
- Asana—a yoga pose of posture that is used to exercise the body and refresh the spirit.
- Kundalini—sexual energy or power based on a Sanskrit word meaning "pool of energy."
- Lingam—the Sanskrit word for *penis* (also known as a "wand of light").
- Shakti—the main female goddess in Hindu Tantra, represents the female essence; she is the creator, sustainer, and destroyer.
- Shiva—the supreme god in Hindu Tantra, represents the male principal; he has control over the movement of time and all material things.
- Yoni—the Sanskrit word for *vagina*.

339. Try Tantric Yoga

Yoga, which means "to join together," is extremely important to Tantra. Yoga brings the focus back to the breath, relieves stress, and allows you to connect with your body. Hatha yoga is the most physically strenuous type and is often practiced by tantric followers, as is kundalini yoga, a type of yoga that places significant emphasis on breathing and postures to achieve different states of consciousness. If you practice yoga you'll likely experience greater flexibility as well as deeper relaxation, and you'll also find that some yoga positions can be used in the bedroom. Yoga can also be amazing in helping you to reach new levels of orgasms, as it helps train you to focus on the moment and connect with your body.

340. Flex Your Muscles in Couples Yoga

One particularly sensual type of yoga is couples yoga. The asanas (or movements) increase your awareness of your partner and help to build a deeper connection between the two of you. Before you begin, sit facing each other with your hands together palm to palm. Maintain eye contact and gently bow to one another as a way to show each other mutual respect and recognize each other's energy. Then begin your poses. Here are some of the more popular movements.

- Happy hug: Stand facing each other with your toes touching. Now hug, releasing yourself into your partner's arms. Take five deep breaths in unison with your partner. Let the air fill your abdomen and then slowly exhale all of it, releasing your tensions, fears, and stress. Take turns rubbing the back of one another for a minute or two.
- Tree together: Stand side by side. Lift your outside leg up and place your foot on your inside leg's thigh above the knee. If you need to, you can support your foot with your hand. Wrap your inside arm around your partner's waist for balance and support. Make your neck as long as you can, stretching it up to the ceiling. Make your legs firm and strong, like roots buried deep in the earth. Breathe in unison and relax into the pose. After taking several deep breaths, switch sides with your partner and repeat the exercise.

- Tantric twist: Sit back to back, with your legs crossed. Make sure that your lower backs are touching, and keep them as close together as possible throughout the exercise. Twist around to your left. Place your left hand on your partner's right knee. Place your right hand on your own left knee. Look behind you and relax your neck and face muscles, pulling firmly on your partner's knee. Take several deep breaths together. Switch directions and repeat.

- Couple's moon triangle: Begin by facing each other, standing with your feet as wide apart as they can comfortably be. Now place your right leg so that it overlaps your partner's left leg, so that you are no longer directly in front of each other but are facing each other somewhat diagonally. Stretch your arms out to either side of your body. Make them as long as you can. Lean over to your right side as your partner does the same. Be sure to keep your hips centered. Tip over like a teapot. Now slide your right hand down your right leg, supporting yourself just above or below the knee, never on the kneecap itself. Extend your other arm straight up toward the ceiling with palm facing inward. You should now be face to face with your partner. Look into each other's eyes. Press your palms together. Hold the position for a while, allowing your energies to flow through each other.

- Couple's lotus pose: Sit in lotus pose, facing each other, with your knees touching those of your partner. Join hands and lay them in the crease between your knees, uniting you both in a continuous flow of energy. Close your eyes and concentrate on the energy between you. Imagine your energies intertwining and mingling. If other thoughts enter your mind, gently let them go. Focus only on your partner's energy. Lose yourself in your partner. This can be an impressive spiritual experience. There is no time limit. Allow yourselves to come out of it when the time feels right.

341. For Him: Love the Lingam Massage

After you and your partner take some time to connect spiritually with the help of couples yoga and through the slow, sensual touching each of you has now finished caressing each other's bodies, offer your partner a lingam massage.

Most often when you're touching his penis, the intent is to arouse him and get him ready for sex, oral sex, or to orgasm with the help of your hand. But in this case, the purpose of a lingam—or penis—massage is to allow your partner to relax and surrender himself to intimate sexual pleasure.

To give one, have your partner lie down on his back and begin to breathe deeply. He should be breathing in through his nose and out through his mouth, and trying to relax his body more fully with each breath. As you massage, look into his eyes, as part of the intent of this massage is to help build spiritual intimacy between you two. Place some oil on the shaft of his penis and his testicles. Massage around the area and up to the pubic bone, move to the perineum, and then begin to massage the shaft itself.

Take your time. Gently take hold of the shaft with one hand, squeeze lightly, move your hand up and down, then slide it off and repeat the same movement with your other hand. Then, place one hand at the base and use the other to massage up and around the penis, and finish each stroke by cupping the glans. When you feel you have thoroughly massaged the penis, move your hand to the perineum and find a small, pea-sized spot. This is the base of the prostate. Press inward delicately as you massage the penis with the other hand. He may get an erection and lose it—then gain it again during the massage, but as the goal is not orgasm, ease off if you feel your partner is nearing ejaculation.

342. Say Yes to the Yoni Massage

As the lingam massage is meant to relax the male, the purpose of the yoni massage is to make the woman feel caressed, adored, and secure so she has the freedom and space to be aroused. If you're a woman, I recommend having your partner read this section so you can lie back and enjoy the massage instead of coaching him through the steps.

Once you have taken the time to awaken your partner's body in a sensual manner, have her lie down on her back and begin to breathe deeply. As you did during the lingam massage, she should breathe in through her nose and out through her mouth, taking special care to let each breath relax her body more than the last.

When she seems fully relaxed, place enough oil on the top of her vulva so that it drips down the outer labia and coats the outside. Take your time and massage around the vulva all the way up to her pubic bone. Then, gently begin stroking the clitoris using circular motions, first clockwise then counterclockwise. When you feel she is ready, slip your middle finger into the vagina and gently feel around the inside, varying the speed and pressure as you go. As she found your "sacred spot" (the prostate gland) during the lingam massage, you're looking to stimulate her "sacred spot" (the G-spot) during the yoni massage. With your palm toward the ceiling, find the G-spot and experiment with speed, pressure, and a variety of strokes. Try circles, back-and-forth motions, and consider inserting your ring finger as well. Continue to look in her eyes as you give the massage, just as she did during the lingam massage, and make sure she is breathing deeply and relaxing into the experience.

If she is enjoying it, you can try placing your thumb on the clitoris and massaging her anus with your pinky. When you have finished the massage, continue to lie with and connect with her until the two of you are ready to move on to orgasm.

343. Pursue the Expansive Orgasm

In Tantric practice, orgasms aren't typically short-lived, anticlimactic experiences that take a long time to reach and then end in one quick moment. Tantric practice often results in expansive orgasms that last much longer than a traditional orgasm. The experience is said to feel like waves of energy coursing through your entire body that cause your spine to undulate and your mind to be completely taken over by the experience. If the regular orgasm is the little death, perhaps the Tantric orgasm is the medium-sized one? To help yourself attain this type of orgasm, you first need to open your mind to the possibility. Once your heart and mind are open, begin to focus on your breath. Practice deep breathing until you are in a very relaxed state. By being aware of your breath, you're going to be more aware of the energy flowing through your body and where you need to work to release blockage.

When you're close to reaching orgasm during Tantric sex (or during regular sex), return to your breath and allow your mind to not focus on any particular thought. Instead, follow the feelings your body is creating within you without judgment or expectation. When you do come, you'll most likely be able to feel the orgasm travel throughout your whole body and turn your orgasm into an incredible full-body experience.

344. Practice Pelvic Lifts and Thrusts

Learning how to move your pelvis in a more fluid manner will improve your abilities in the bedroom and may help improve your orgasms. You can practice these pelvic exercises alone or with your partner. Personally, I'd recommend doing them alone, as they do look awfully silly. That said, strengthening your hips and relaxing your hip flexors will improve your movements in the bedroom, so this is one case where feeling silly is worth it.

Put on some hip-shaking music and begin by thrusting your hips from front to back while standing up. Start out slowly, focusing on the hips only while keeping your upper body still and steady. Once you've isolated the hips, start moving them in different directions, which you can later try out when you're having sex.

Similar to pelvic thrusts are pelvic lifts. These are practiced by lying on your back on the floor with your knees up. When you're in this position, lift your hips as high as you can off the floor and hold them in this position for several seconds. This also works your butt and abdominal muscles, so you're not only helping your sex life, you're getting toned while doing it.

345. Make Your Meditation Orgasmic

Recently, a new practice known as orgasmic meditation has begun to pop up across the country through a group known as OneTaste. Though the group shares some common beliefs with Tantra, their purpose is to create a more embodied sense of self and a feeling of wholeness through mindful sexuality and meditation. To attempt orgasmic meditation with your partner, have him slowly stroke your clitoris with his index finger while both of you focus your complete awareness on that part of your body with no intention of taking the sexual act to the next level. You may come many times during this meditation, and as you and your partner develop your meditative skills, followers of the practice claim that both partners can achieve a long-lasting, full-body orgasm.

346. Explore the Ancient Sex Manuals

It isn't just our current—and some might say sex-obsessed—culture that is interested in what goes on between the sheets. For centuries, humans have been fascinated with sex and how they can improve their performance. Considering that just centuries ago many couples had no sexual experiences prior to their marriage, these pillow books were helpful, eye-opening (and sometimes beautifully illustrated) guides that helped these couples explore their sexuality and taught them ways in which they could pleasure their new partner. Even though this sort of experience is not what most of us confront today, these books still have much to offer in helping you discover new paths to orgasm.

347. Read the Kama Sutra

Around A.D. 350, scholar Mallanga Vatsyayana penned the *Kama Sutra*, the first known written work to focus on the art of lovemaking. Following Sir Richard Burton's translation of it into English in the 1800s, it became—and may still be—the world's most popular book on sex. In fact, many of the sex positions included in this book are from or influenced by the *Kama Sutra*. But the ancient text is much more than just a guide to great sexual positions. It's actually based on two sets of Sixty-Four Arts, only one of which deals with sex and foreplay. The other set discusses the arts and skills Vatsyayana felt were necessary for a person to become well-rounded. These include how to find a wife, what to do about prostitutes, and how to improve your sexual prowess.

348. Read the Ishimpo

Though this thirty-volume book written between the eighth and twelfth centuries in Japan is really a medical text that covers everything from dermatology to internal medicine, one of the volumes does tackle the complicated subject of human sexuality. The tome is impressive for many reasons, including the fact that it managed to preserve some of the Taoist sex manuals from the Han through Tang dynasties. But perhaps my favorite part of that section of the book is the part that states that sex between men and women is the life force controlling the universe and making love is what keeps Earth circling the heavens. In the writer's mind, love really did make the world go round.

349. Check Out the Ananga Ranga

Whereas the *Kama Sutra* was all the rage after the sixth century in India, this manual instructed later generations of the sexually curious when it was written in the sixteenth century. It included everything from morals and seduction techniques to sexual spells, rituals, and, of course, positions. The text was also one of the first documented promoters of using the Kegel exercise as a way for a woman to strengthen her pelvic floor and heighten her orgasm.

350. Walk Through The Perfumed Garden

Another book written in the sixteenth century was *The Perfumed Garden*, penned in Arabia. Though written with a male audience in mind, it doesn't just focus on the man's pleasure. Instead, it was very ahead of its time, as it suggested that men discover what their women enjoy and ask their lovers for help on how to give them pleasure. In addition to this wise guidance, it taught the readers what the male and female genitals looked like and how to connect pleasure and sexuality to spirituality.

351. Explore the Secrets of the Jade Bed Chamber

This ancient Chinese manual, written during the Han dynasty in the third century, centered around sexuality and sensuality and includes similar topics as the other guides I've mentioned, such as relationship and courting counseling, sexual positions, and ways to improve potency. As with Tantra, the book also provides its own names for the male and female genitalia. In the book, the penis is known as the Jade Stalk while the vagina is called the Jade Garden.

352. Indulge in the Ars Amatoria

One final early manuscript focused on love and sex was written by the Latin poet Ovid around 1 B.C. *Ars Amatoria* (translated from the Latin to mean "The Art of Love") is a poem in three parts that describes where to find women worth having sex with, how to seduce them, and how to keep other men from running away with them. Many of his teachings, from the sex positions to his reminders to men not to forget their lover's birthday, can still be used today. Though if you're searching for something that's on the more ribald side, this literary work isn't going to satisfy your craving.

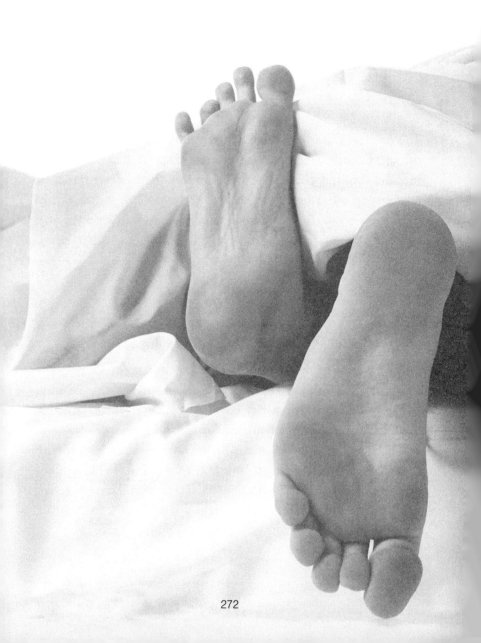

CHAPTER TWENTY-ONE

Improve Your Orgasms Again and Again and . . .

353. Enhance Your Orgasm

By this point, I hope that through all the tips, techniques, ideas, and positions I've suggested, you've had some impressive orgasms and found ways to clear out those obstacles that have gotten in your way in the past. Perhaps you finally even experienced your first orgasm! Or you found a position that is now your new go-to. In these last few tips, I want to give you a couple final ideas you can integrate to enhance your orgasms. Great work getting here, and best of luck as you go back to the bedroom armed with your new knowledge. Make sure you always focus on improving what you like, rather than settling for any ol' orgasm that comes about. Switch up your hand placement, or reduce the speed of the vibrations—any little alteration can make a huge difference. Try it as many different ways as you can think of!

354. Focus on the Journey

Have you ever heard someone talk about how the journey is more important than the destination? Orgasms fit into that category as well. That's because even if you have a great orgasm, if the circumstances surrounding it are mediocre—or even bad or downright dull—it's likely you'll remember the ho-hum or disconnected sex and not the climax that made your head spin 'round. So unless it's an intentional quickie brought on by some serious animalistic passion, don't rush up the mountain of lovemaking just so you can reach the top.

355. Slow Down

When the intention in the bedroom is to focus on the pathway to orgasm instead of just the climax, it's easier to slow down and take time with each movement. This type of pace builds sexual tension as well as a deeper connection with your partner, which can improve the orgasm when it comes. When you're in bed with your man, make it a point during some of your lovemaking sessions to build very close to the point of no return, then back off again a few times until you are ready to finish the journey together. When you do, you may find the orgasm you experience to be more powerful than the one you would have had if you'd succumbed to your desire for instant gratification.

356. Learn to Enjoy Yourself!

American culture is at war with itself when it comes to sex. On the one hand, advertisers use sex to entice the public to buy pretty much anything, be it a car or a hamburger. But when it comes to talking openly about sex or being happy with the bodies we're in, we're lost. Did you know that about 26 percent of American woman report that they have never experienced an orgasm?! That's a completely unreasonable number and one we should work to whittle down. In the meantime, you can work on your own acceptance of your sexuality, your body, and the body of your partner. Revisit some of the chapters within this book to help you along that path, and, unless you're practicing exploring each other's bodies in the complete darkness as a way to enhance your sex life, light some candles so you can practice admiring each other!

357. Breathe with Your Partner

Getting to the edge of orgasm and then just not making it there can be extremely frustrating. One way to help yourself when you're feeling stuck is by *breathing*. "But I *am* breathing!" you say. Uh-huh. Well, even if you're not turning blue, next time you're having trouble climaxing, put some focus on your breath—*not the orgasm*—and take slow, deep, full-body breaths. For some tips on how to breathe, return to the sections of the book where I discuss yoga and Tantra, as both of those practices focus on connecting with your mind and spirit as well as with your body. The idea is to experience sex as a pleasurable activity on its own instead of treating it as a means to an end. By breathing and relaxing, you take some pressure off of the orgasm and put it into the journey to get there. By doing so, you're probably going to have to work back up to the point where you're about to come, but when you reach that point again in this more relaxed state, you'll be more likely to reach the climax instead of fall off the cliff.

358. Hold Your Breath

I realize that I just told you to breathe if you're having trouble reaching orgasm. And for most people, holding their breath and tensing their body actually minimizes the power of an orgasm. But if you don't have trouble coming, you could make your orgasms more powerful by holding your breath. Instead of using a dangerous device like a tie or something else that you may accidentally choke yourself with when you climax, simply hold your breath and don't let go until your orgasm has passed. It won't take too many tries before you find out whether taking full breaths or holding your breath when you're close to orgasm is more effective at getting you there.

359. Reach Orgasm Simultaneously

Orgasms are great on their own, but even better when they come in pairs. And in this case, I don't mean multiple. I mean coming with your partner at the same time. When you and your man are able to reach climax at the same time, it's an amazing way to connect. But it can also heighten the orgasm itself, as each of you could find yourself getting more turned on as the other starts to move their hips and contract their penis (or in your case, your vagina) in a way that's purely primal. Then, when you both get there, you can collapse into each other's arms in postecstasy bliss.

360. Have Unprotected Sex

Safe sex is important, as it can help prevent the transmission of STIs. But if you're in a faithful, committed relationship and are either on hormonal birth control or are trying to get pregnant, there's nothing like the feeling of having your lover ejaculate inside of you. It's possibly the only way to make even the best orgasm feel better. And did you know that women have been known to have spontaneous orgasms when their bodies recognize that the guy has deposited semen in their vagina? Thanks, biology!

361. Orgasm on Your Partner

Though most of this book has been devoted to finding new ways of achieving great orgasms, *where* you orgasm is also important. Coming inside of your partner—or having them come inside of you—is very intimate and intense. But it can also be fun to come on your partner or for him to give you a pearl necklace. Many men love watching their own money shot of sperm land on top of their partner's breasts, face, tummy, or lower back. Master female ejaculation and you can return the favor!

362. Do It More Than Once

Though it takes some training for women to experience external ejaculation, women do have the advantage of being able to experience multiple orgasms relatively easily. There are two types of multiple orgasms: sequential and serial. Sequential orgasms are those that occur spaced out from each other, while serial orgasms can happen within mere seconds of the last one, so they feel more like one continuous orgasm.

363. Experience Multiple Orgasms

If, like most women, you rely on your clitoris as your primary gateway to orgasm, most likely you will want to give this organ a reprieve after the first orgasm and focus on stimulating other erogenous zones, or continue enjoying penetration without direct stimulation of the clitoris. But if you want to achieve a strong sequential or serial orgasm, try to push past the feeling that your clitoris is too sensitive for continued contact and ask your partner to keep up the motion that got you going in the first place.

364. Help Him to Achieve Multiple Orgasms

Most men have a much harder time experiencing multiple orgasms than women do because they have a longer refractory period. Few men can ejaculate, get stimulated, and then ejaculate again within one sexual episode. But there is a way to do it. It all goes back to those Kegel exercises you learned earlier in the book. By strengthening and gaining control of the PC muscle, he'll just need to squeeze it hard as soon as he begins having an orgasm to prevent ejaculation but allow the rush of orgasm to flood through his body. This will allow him to maintain an erection and come again and again until he's ready to ejaculate.

365. Don't Fake It

You've read, you've tried new positions, you've practiced the techniques I've suggested. Face it: you've worked hard to learn how to have a great orgasm! Here's the most important thing you need to know: Don't fake your orgasm. Not much, if any, good can come from moaning when you're not turned on and pretending to reach climax when your partner isn't getting you there. All you're doing is inflating an undeserving ego. If your partner can't get you off—and he may not be able to every time you're in bed together—it's more important that the two of you figure out what's going on and solve the issue instead of sticking your heads in the sand. So, unless you want your partner to misunderstand what works for you, lay off the acting until Hollywood calls!

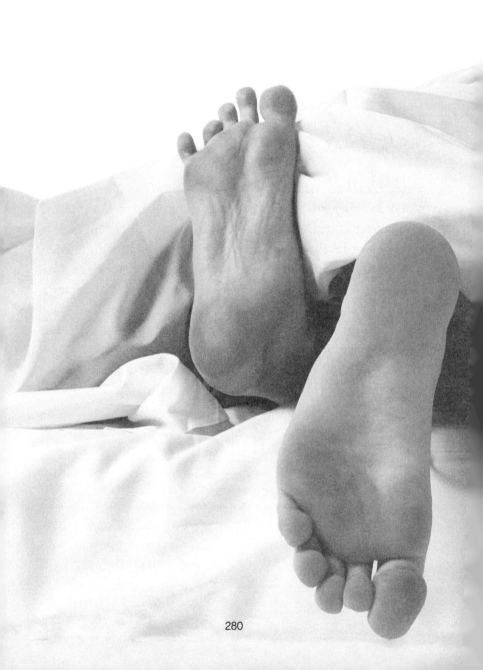

Index